Critical Nursing Care of the Client with Cancer

Critical Nursing Care of the Client with Cancer

Cynthia C. Chernecky, M.N., R.N.
Assistant Professor
Clinical Specialist in Oncology Nursing
College of Nursing
Clemson University
Clemson, South Carolina

Priscilla W. Ramsey, M.S., R.N., C.S.
Assistant Professor
Clinical Specialist in Medical-Surgical Nursing
College of Nursing
Clemson University
Clemson, South Carolina

Contributing Author:
Priscilla M. Kline, M.S.N., R.N.
Assistant Professor
Private Psychiatric-Mental Health Nursing Practice
in Individual and Family Therapy
College of Nursing
Clemson University
Clemson, South Carolina

APPLETON-CENTURY-CROFTS/Norwalk, Connecticut

ISBN 0-8385-1243-7

84 85 86 87 88 89 / 10 9 8 7 6 5 4 3 2 1

Prentice-Hall International, Inc., London
Prentice-Hall of Australia, Pty. Ltd., Sydney
Prentice-Hall Canada, Inc.
Prentice-Hall of India Private Limited, New Delhi
Prentice-Hall of Japan, Inc., Tokyo
Prentice-Hall of Southeast Asia (Pte.) Ltd., Singapore
Whitehall Books Ltd., Wellington, New Zealand
Editora Prentice-Hall do Brasil Ltda., Rio de Janeiro

Library of Congress Cataloging in Publication Data

Chernecky, Cynthia C.
   Critical nursing care of the client with cancer.

   Includes index.
   1. Cancer—Nursing. 2. Intensive care nursing.
I. Ramsey, Priscilla W. II. Kline, Priscilla M.
III. Title. [DNLM: 1. Critical Care—nurses' instruction.
2. Neoplasms—nursing. WY 156 C521c]
RC266.C48 1984   610.73'698   84-11051
ISBN 0-8385-1243-7

PRINTED IN THE UNITED STATES OF AMERICA

The development of this book could not have occurred without the love, encouragement, and wisdom of my family—my mother Olga, my late father Edward, and my brother Richard.
I owe a great deal to my mentors, who have given unsparingly and unselfishly of their time and knowledge: Jadwiga Goclowski, R.N., M.S.N.; Joyce M. Yasko, R.N., Ph.D.; Mary Ann Kelly, R.N., Ed.D.; and Claire Gulino, R.N., Ed.D.

Cynthia C. (Cinda) Chernecky

To my son Jack, whose enthusiasm, love, and optimism provides me the courage to attempt yet another challenge, to the critical care and oncology staff nurses, who never seem to exhaust their ability to care, endure, and strive for excellence, and to Frances Storlie, R.N., Ph.D., who convinced me I could write, I dedicate this book.

Priscilla W. Ramsey

Contents

Foreword

Twenty years ago a book devoted to the critical and emergency care of the cancer client would have appeared unnecessary. Surgery was the primary therapy then, with only limited use of radiation and occasional drug treatments. Clients who became critically ill rarely survived, because their tumor was beyond control and information about how to sustain clients was only beginning to be discovered.

Among science's greatest achievements is the drastic reversal of this situation. Cancer survival statistics have improved to the point that today half of all cancer clients can be cured using current knowledge of early diagnosis and therapy.

The therapies themselves have changed. Radiation therapy and the use of anticancer drugs have expanded rapidly. Surgery no longer is the sole treatment. Many tumors are treated using multimodality strategies. This quantum leap in anticancer therapy occurred concurrently with the expansion of knowledge about how cancer acts. The propensity for small, often undetectable numbers of cancer cells to multiply and kill the client has demanded aggressive treatment that can have devastating effects on normal as well as tumor cells. Consequently, clients can become acutely ill due to either the therapy or the tumor. Moreover, the incidence of acute episodes among cancer clients has increased and will continue to increase as new treatments are developed.

It is now known that clients who weather the storm of a critical episode often experience an improvement in their chance of survival or quality of life or both. Cancer, then, approaches a chronic illness with acute phases rather than a disease with a short life trajectory. Recognizing this phenomenon means that nurses and other health professionals must be astute at detecting impending critical episodes and providing sophisticated interventions to foster client survival.

The authors, by combining their critical care expertise and extensive cancer knowledge, have developed an exceptional resource for guiding nurses in the development of relevant care for patients during emergency or critical episodes. The chapters in this book are organized according to physiologic alterations, which enables the reader to locate specific material quickly. Furthermore, each chapter is comprehensive, which eliminates time-consuming cross-referencing exercises. The authors present each topic in a logical sequence from concise description of the pathophysiologic mechanism to nursing diagnoses and practical intervention guides.

Critical Nursing Care of the Client with Cancer reflects the newest dimension in cancer care, the critical care episode. It warrants inclusion in both critical care and cancer nursing collections.

Anne R. Bavier, R.N., M.N.
Associate Professor and Coordinator Cancer Specialty
Yale University School of Nursing
New Haven, Connecticut

Preface

Critical nursing care of the client with cancer requires comprehensive nursing knowledge that includes nursing theory, cellular physiobiochemistry, neoplastic pathophysiology, radiotherapy, antineoplastic pharmacotherapeutics, and genetic, immunologic, and epidemiologic theories. The client with cancer is at potential risk for serious and often life-threatening complications resulting from the pathologic processes of cancer and the iatrotechnology involved in the treatment of cancer. Oncology-related complications demand immediate recognition and effective management in order to avert irreversible trauma and jeopardy to life.

The main purpose in writing this book is to present a primary reference of potential problems requiring immediate intervention specific to the client with cancer. Although the emphasis is nursing-directed, any health care professional could benefit from its contents in anticipating complications and planning care. This text is intended for use on oncology units, critical care units, and in the classroom. It can also be used as a standard in evaluating care for institutional audit and in planning for the development of an oncology unit. This book is based on the combined experiences of the authors in oncology, critical care, and psychiatric/mental-health nursing.

The second purpose in undertaking this project is to demonstrate the importance of collaboration between nursing specialties in order to improve the quality and outcome of nursing care.

The third reason is to stimulate interest in oncology nursing—nursing the client with cancer—among students and practitioners of nursing. Specialization is as essential in nursing as it is in other disciplines, and the authors feel that oncology nursing is an exciting and rewarding field. Cancer research is producing new information more rapidly than we are able to read it. Some have predicted that a cancer cure will be among the next major scientific breakthroughs. Far from the depressing prognosis of a decade ago, clients experiencing cancer today have more alternative therapies than ever before. The survival rate of clients with cancer is progressively increasing because of recent aggressive educational programs for early detection, aggressive surgical, chemotherapeutic, and radiological therapies, and aggressive treatment of cancer and therapy induced life-threatening complications.

The final purpose of this book is to present critical nursing care of the client with cancer within the framework of professional nursing, including nursing concepts, nursing processes, and nursing diagnoses. The role of the professional nurse in implementing holistic care for the client is requiring more and more professional, technical, and intellectual expertise. Theories involving crisis, stress, coping mechanisms, family, adaptation, and death and dying are some components of these approaches.

The book is divided into ten parts according to concepts reflecting a contemporary emphasis in nursing education. Each chapter begins with a brief discussion and definition of the oncological problem describing the anatomical, physiological, or biochemical component in relation to the neoplastic process. The most common causative factors of each problem are listed according to priority of causation. Additional factors are also listed and include conditions or diseases unrelated to cancer that could precipitate the specified complication separately or in combination with the neoplasm.

The assessment data are placed in order according to priority and provide the basis for making the nursing diagnosis. Although the use of nursing diagnoses is still somewhat controversial, it is the opinion of the authors that nursing diagnoses represent professional expertise in logically organizing assessment data and planning care and are essential to nursing practice. Most of the nursing diagnoses in this book list multiple etiologies and results based on the data.

Acknowledgments

Our deep appreciation to Nancy Carls, whose expert typing and skillful handling of the manuscript was essential to its completion. Her patience, dedication, and struggle during the pressures of the final weeks deserve particular praise and commendation. Nancy has sworn off typing another manuscript, especially since this one was typed during her transition from single-vision to bifocal glasses.

Special thanks to Dr. Mary Lohr, Dean and Professor of Clemson University's College of Nursing, for providing us the freedom in our professional environment that allowed the creation of ideas for this book.

Thanks also to the publishing company of Appleton-Century-Crofts for making this book possible, and especially to Marion Kalstein, Editor, for her cooperation and enthusiasm, and Daniel Payne, Production Editor, for his expertise.

Our deepest gratitude to Ann Bavier, R.N., M.N., Jo Anne Peter, R.N., M.S., Ann W. Baxter, Ph.D., Karen B. Heusinkueld, R.N., Ph.D., and Nancy Kane, R.N., M.S. for their review of the manuscript.

Cynthia C. Chernecky
Priscilla W. Ramsey

Introduction

Critical Nursing Care of the Client with Cancer was designed to be used by the nurse in two ways: first, to anticipate possible complications in the adult client with a specific cancer, and second, to assist the nurse in identifying complications occurring in the adult client based on the presenting data. Anticipatory planning is a process by which the nurse responds to these three questions:

1. What are the possible complications that could occur in the client with a specific cancer?
2. How would the nurse recognize the onset of a related complication?
3. What interventions should the nurse take?

The first question can be answered by utilizing the Potential Problem List (p. xvii) as a guide in identifying the most common complications of specific cancers. It was developed after reviewing the current literature, surveying practitioners in oncology, and drawing on our own experiences. Its function is to provide an immediate reference for the nurse when the client is admitted to the health care facility. The Potential Problem List is in order for each cancer category according to the frequency of occurrence.

The second question can be answered by referring to the Assessment Data List in each chapter. This list is ordered according to which sign(s) or symptom(s) the client would *most likely* exhibit first. The Assessment Data List was derived from literature, research, experience, or inference based on the pathophysiologic processes. The reader must realize, however, that there will always be individual differences, and the total picture must be considered.

The third question can be answered by utilizing the section on Nursing Interventions in each chapter. Nursing interventions are categorized as "monitoring" or "change." Monitoring interventions are all those requiring objective and subjective data gathering techniques which determine the status of the client. Monitoring interventions determine change interventions, which are nursing actions assisting in the prevention or treatment of oncological complications. Change interventions are also those considered in the evaluation process.

Nursing interventions are further categorized as either "independent" or "interdependent." Independent nursing interventions are those actions based solely on nursing decisions, and interdependent interventions are those nursing actions influenced by medical intervention and/or interventions from other health care professionals. Nursing interventions are ordered in relation to the primary nursing diagnosis. Basic nursing actions are not included unless a specific modification is required.

Many areas in nursing practice are not clearly defined as specific to the domain of the nurse or the domain of the physician. For example, although in some institutions applying oxygen at 2 L/min by nasal cannula or starting D5W IV at KVO require a physician's authorization, others consider these as standard practice based on the decision of the professional nurse. We are attempting to address these grey areas in a rational rather than an emotional way, although we do not expect to find complete agreement in each instance.

Potential Problem List
for the Client With
Primary or Metastatic Cancer

Under each heading—representing a type of cancer or a cancer problem area—the potential problems are listed in order according to frequency of occurrence. Each problem is treated separately in its own chapter. For quick reference, the page numbers have also been listed.

BLADDER/KIDNEY

Obstructive Uropathy / 235
Pathologic Fractures / 179
Hypercalcemia / 1
Spinal Cord Compression / 195
Amyloidosis / 217

BREAST

Reactive Depression / 265
Pathologic Fractures / 179
Postmastectomy Lymphedema / 52
Hypercalcemia / 1
Intracerebral Metastasis / 187
Spinal Cord Compression / 195
Superior Vena Cava Syndrome / 81
Pleural Effusion / 129
Meningeal Carcinomatosis / 202
Neoplastic Pericardial Effusion and
  Tamponade / 88
Constrictive Pericarditis / 95
Thrombophlebitis / 106
Suicidal Ideation / 272
Disseminated Intravascular
  Coagulation / 67

CENTRAL NERVOUS SYSTEM

Intracerebral Metastasis / 187
Reactive Depression / 265
Spinal Cord Compression / 195
Meningeal Carcinomatosis / 202
Suicidal Ideation / 272

CERVIX/UTERINE

Thrombocytopenia / 61
Obstructive Uropathy / 235

CHEMOTHERAPY

Hyperuricemia / 229
Cardiomyopathy / 100
Neutropenic and Nonneutropenic
  Sepsis / 147
Cell-Mediated Immunity
  Impairment / 165
Endogenous Hemorrhagic
  Gastritis / 73
Thrombocytopenia / 61
Potential Complications of Total
  Parenteral Nutrition / 255

LUNG

Pleural Effusion / 129
Secretion of Inappropriate
   Antidiuretic Hormone / 46
Spontaneous Pneumothorax / 123
Radiation Pneumonitis / 142
Pathologic Fractures / 179
Intracerebral Metastasis / 187
Superior Vena Cava Syndrome
   (Oat Cell Carcinoma) / 81
Hypomagnesemia (Oat Cell
   Carcinoma) / 27
Hyponatremia / 14
Thrombophlebitis / 106
Pulmonary Embolism / 135
Airway Obstruction / 113
Spinal Cord Compression / 195
Disseminated Intravascular
   Coagulation / 67

LYMPHOMA see
Hodgkin's/Lymphoma

MELANOMA

Intracerebral Metastasis / 187
Spinal Cord Compression / 195
Pericardial Effusion and
   Tamponade / 88
Endogenous Hemorrhagic
   Gastritis / 73
Disseminated Intravascular
   Coagulation / 67
Meningeal Carcinomatosis / 202
Constrictive Pericarditis / 95
Small Bowel Obstruction / 243

MULTIPLE MYELOMA

Amyloidosis / 217
Hypercalcemia / 1
Hypophosphatemia / 8
Cell-Mediated Immunity
   Impairment / 165
Hyperuricemia / 229
Pathologic Fractures / 179

MULTIPLE MYELOMA (cont.)

Reactive Depression / 265
Aspiration Pneumonia / 118
Hypokalemia / 20
Hyponatremia / 14
Spinal Cord Compression / 195
Obstructive Uropathy / 235

NECK see Head/Neck

OVARY

Hypomagnesemia / 27
Pleural Effusion / 129
Thrombophlebitis / 106
Pathologic Fractures / 179
Secretion of Inappropriate Antidiuretic
   Hormone / 46
Hypercalcemia / 1
Disseminated Intravascular
   Coagulation / 67
Hyponatremia / 14
Reactive Depression / 265
Obstructive Uropathy / 235
Constrictive Pericarditis / 95
Small Bowel Obstruction / 243

PANCREAS

Secretion of Inappropriate Antidiuretic
   Hormone / 46
Hypokalemia / 20
Pulmonary Embolism / 135
Malabsorption Syndrome / 249
Thrombophlebitis / 106
Hyponatremia / 14
Complications of Total Parenteral
   Nutrition / 255
Reactive Depression / 265
Pathologic Fractures / 179
Hypercalcemia / 1
Disseminated Intravascular
   Coagulation / 67
Small Bowel Obstruction / 243
Obstructive Uropathy / 235
Meningeal Carcinomatosis / 202

Critical Nursing
Care of the
Client with Cancer

PART I
FLUID AND ELECTROLYTE BALANCE

1. Hypercalcemia

DEFINITION AND CAUSATIVE FACTORS

Hypercalcemia in the client with cancer occurs when the serum concentration of calcium exceeds 11 mg/dl; the normal range is 8.5 to 10.5 mg/dl. The abnormal release of calcium is caused by several bone resorptive (demineralization) mechanisms: bone destruction by metastasis, prolonged immobilization, high concentrations of parathyroid hormone (PTH) found in some tumors, and two potent resorptive substances, prostaglandins and osteoclast activating factor (OAF), found in cancer clients with hypercalcemia.

Normally, calcium is regulated by feedback mechanisms of PTH (parathyroid), 1,25 dioxycholecalciferol (kidney), and calcitonin (thyroid). When calcium levels are low, PTH stimulates bone to release calcium and phosphorus, activating the kidneys to convert a vitamin D metabolite to 1,25 dioxycholecalciferol which increases the absorption of calcium through the gastrointestinal (GI) tract. PTH also regulates excretion or reabsorption of calcium in the kidneys. Calcitonin inhibits these processes when calcium concentrations are elevated or within normal range. Only 1% of the total body calcium is found in blood; 50% of the total body calcium is protein bound and the other 50% is ionized. The relationship of calcium and phosphorus is inversely proportional; when one ion is increased, the other is decreased. Calcium has many functions in the body: bone calcification and teeth formation, growth, blood clotting (factor I), catalyst for several biological reactions including absorption of vitamin B_{12}, maintenance of function of cell membranes, regulation of muscle contraction, and transmission of nerve impulses.

Ten to twenty percent of all clients with cancer will develop hypercalcemia, and of those with metastatic breast cancer or multiple myeloma, the incidence is 40 to 50%. Other corresponding cancers include: multiple myeloma, leukemia, lymphoma, lung, kidney, head and neck, cervix, neuroblastoma, ovary, pancreas, and bladder. Hypophosphatemia, renal failure, prolonged immobility, parathyroid deficiency, mithramycin chemotherapy, and digitalis toxicity are additional causes.

ASSESSMENT DATA

- Serum calcium greater than 12.0 mg/dl
- Polyuria—early sign
- Polydipsia
- Dehydration—can be severe
- Renal calculi
- Fatigue and profound muscle weakness
- Hyporeflexia of deep tendon reflexes
- Altered perception and behavior
- Anorexia, nausea, and vomiting
- Paralytic ileus
- Peptic ulcer
- Pruritis
- Constipation
- Arrhythmias
- Mithramycin chemotherapy
- Hypophosphatemia
- Hypokalemia
- Digitalis toxicity
- Bone pain
- Increased alkaline phosphatase
- Stupor and coma—late sign
- Renal failure—late sign

EKG Changes

- Short QT interval with characteristic coved ST junction
- Prolonged PR interval
- If serum calcium greater than 16 mg/dl QT interval lengthens and T wave widens
- With digitalis toxicity any arrhythmia or A-V block or bradycardia

NURSING DIAGNOSES

Fluid volume deficit, related to dehydration and polyuria, resulting from an increased serum calcium concentration.

Associated Nursing Diagnoses

1. Alteration in cardiac output, decreased, related to a potential for digitalis toxicity caused by excessive serum calcium levels resulting in arrhythmias.

RATIONALE

Concentrating ability of renal tubules is decreased.

Calcium enhances the action of digitalis causing bradycardia–arrhythmias.

2. Potential for physical injury, related to bone destruction and possible pathological fractures resulting from increased serum calcium levels.

Increased PTH or increased absorption of calcium (multiple myeloma) increases bone demineralization.

3. Decreased activity tolerance, related to fatigue and muscular weakness, resulting from a serum calcium excess.

Decreased neuronal permeability.

4. Impaired thought processes, related to alterations in awareness, orientation, and behavior, resulting from hypercalcemia.

Decreased neuronal permeability.

5. Alteration in nutrition, less than body requirements, related to anorexia, nausea, and vomiting resulting from hypercalcemia.

Decreased neuronal permeability.

NURSING INTERVENTIONS

Monitoring–Independent

1. Hourly I and O and calculate I/O ratio for fluid balance q 8 and 24 hr.
2. Urine specific gravity q 4 to 8 hr.
3. BP, heart rate, respirations q 2 hr.
4. Temperature q 4 hr.
5. Assess LOC q 4 to 8 hr and record changes in awareness, orientation, and behavior.
6. Assess cardiac rhythm strip for changes in PR interval, ST junction, and T wave q 1 to 2 hr with increasing serum calcium levels.
7. Assess client's tolerance for activity and subjective indications of fatigue and weakness q 4 hr.
8. Test deep tendon reflexes q 8 hr by tapping biceps, triceps, patellae, and Achilles tendon, and record onset of decreased response.
9. Assess client for flank pain (renal calculi), bone pain (demineralization or pathological fractures), and abdominal pain (ileus) with each client contact.
10. Strain all urine for calculi.
11. Assess skin color, temperature, moisture, turgor, and itching q 4 to 8 hr.

12. Assess for thirst, nausea, vomiting with each client contact.
13. Auscultate bowel sounds in all 4 quadrants q 8 hr and record onset of changes in pitch and frequency. Palpate for abdominal rigidity.
14. Assess cardiac rhythm for arrhythmia and A-V block continuously with serum calcium levels greater than 11 mg/dl.
15. Determine pH of NG secretions (if applicable) q 4 to 8 hr (hypercalcemia causes an increased acid secretion).
16. Hemocult all stools and emesis.
17. Weigh q AM before breakfast and record.
18. Auscultate heart sounds in 4 valvular sites q 8 hr and record onset of extra heart sounds.
19. Auscultate breath sounds in all lung fields q 8 hr and record onset of adventitious sounds.

Monitoring–Interdependent

1. Assess results of laboratory data when available and compare to previous and normal values.
   Serum Calcium: 8.5 to 10.5 mg/dl
   Serum Sodium: 135 to 145 mEq/L
   Serum Potassium: 3.5 to 5.0 mEq/L
   Serum Chloride: 100 to 106 mEq/L
   Alkaline Phosphatase: 13 to 39 IU
   Phosphorus: 3.0 to 4.5 mg/dl
   Serum Immunoreactive Parathormone (iPTH): lower than serum calcium level when due to cancer
   Digoxin Level: therapeutic range = 0.8 to 1.9 ng/ml
   BUN: 8 to 25 mg/dl
   Creatinine: 0.6 to 1.5 mg/dl
   Urine Specific Gravity: 1.015 to 1.025
   Urine Calcium: 150 mg/25 hr or less
2. Assess IV site for redness, pain, swelling q 4 to 8 hr.
3. Assess client for hypocalcemia after initiation of therapy.
   Serum calcium levels less than 8.5 mg/dl
   Positive Chvostek and Trousseau signs
   Tetany

Change–Independent

1. Maintain bedrest and minimize activity with serum calcium levels greater than 11.0 mg/dl.

2. Offer fluids to 120 ml q 1 hr while awake, alternating with juice and water, if tolerated.

3. Apply ice collar to neck with onset of nausea.

4. Institute all safety measures by elevating side rails, padding if client restless or disoriented, and placing all personal articles and call light within easy reach.

5. Reorient to person, time, place, and reason for hospitalization with each contact if client confused or disoriented.

6. Position for maximum comfort and protection of fragile bones.

7. Mouth care q 4 hr, after each vomiting episode, and before meals using appropriate oral antiseptic that is refreshing without tasting too sweet. Once a day, clean teeth with a mixture of H_2O_2 and baking soda to neutralize oral acid and remove plaque.

8. Passive ROME to all major joints while on bedrest q 4 hr.

9. Turn, cough, deep breathe q 2 hr while on bedrest.

10. Back care q 4 hr while on bedrest and massage all bony prominences with lotion.

11. Institute gradual increase in activity when client can tolerate it or when prescribed by physician.

12. O_2 at 2 L/min by nasal cannula if SOB occurs.

13. Assist client to perform ADLs and maintain judicious independence and control over self and environment within physical limitations.

14. Explain condition and progress to client and family with each contact. Assist them to ask questions and express concerns of the present and the future.

15. Include family members in plan of care and allow them to participate if mutually beneficial.

Change–Interdependent

1. Consult with dietitian about diet low in calcium (limited milk, cheese, collards, turnip greens, cabbage, soybean), high in potassium (muscle meats, dried and fresh fruits, tomatoes, potatoes), high in magnesium (whole grains, spinach, beef), or as prescribed by physician.

2. Medicate appropriately for pain, emesis, or arrhythmia as prescribed and assess effect in 1 to 20 min.

3. Normal saline at KVO or as prescribed.

4. Notify physician if:
   Serum calcium greater than 11 mg/dl or less than 8.5 mg/dl after initiation of therapy. Levels less than 8.0 mg/dl, arrhythmia onset, or severe hypotension.

Serum sodium greater than 145 mEq/L or less than 135 mEq/L.

Serum potassium greater than 6 mEq/L

and BUN greater than 25 mg/dl.

and weight greater than 4 pound gain.

and creatinine greater than 2 mg/dl (indicating impending renal failure).

Digoxin level greater than 2.0 ng/ml

EKG changes or arrhythmia indicating hypercalcemia.

Systolic blood pressure less than 90 torr.

Sudden onset of bone, abdominal, or flank pain.

High pitched, absent, or diminished bowel sounds.

Positive stool or emesis hemocult.

5. Anticipate the physician to prescribe:

IV normal saline 3 to 5 L/24 hr to rehydrate and to facilitate excretion of excess calcium.

Lasix: 80 to 100 mg q 1 to 2 hr if hypercalcemia severe. Calcium and sodium have similar urinary excretory mechanisms; if sodium is eliminated by the action of Lasix, so will calcium.

IV Inorganic Phosphates: fastest method of reducing serum calcium levels and can be very rapid causing calcium phosphate salt deposit in bone. Oral route only for clients in renal failure (Neutraphos).

Steroids (Prednisone): 300 to 400 mg/24 hr to increase excretion of calcium.

Mithramycin: 12.5 to 25 micrograms/kg to directly inhibit bone resorption but side effects include thrombocytopenia, hypotension, and renal damage.

Indomethacin: to inhibit prostaglandin synthesis.

Calcitonin: 2 to 8 MRC units/kg to inhibit bone resorption, but rarely used.

Decrease in dosage of estrogens, androgens, or progestins for clients being treated for breast cancer (hypercalcemia is exacerbated by these compounds).

BIBLIOGRAPHY

Avioli, L.V. Calcitonin therapy for bone disease and hypercalcemia. Archives of Internal Medicine, 142, 1982, 2076–2079 (Editorial).

Brayko, C.M. and Doll, D.C. Squamous cell carcinoma of the pancreas associated with hypercalcemia. Gastroenterology, 83, 1982, 1297–1299.

Britton, D. and Yasko, J.M. Hypercalcemia. In J.M. Yasko (ed.), Guidelines for Cancer Care—Symptom Management. Virginia: Reston, 1983.

Bull, F.E. Hypercalcemia in cancer. In J. Yarbro and R. Bornstein (eds.), *Oncologic Emergencies*. New York: Grune and Stratton, 1981.

Corbett, J.V. *Laboratory tests in nursing practice*. Norwalk, Connecticut: Appleton-Century-Crofts, 1982.

Delamore, I.W. Hypercalcemia and myeloma: Clinical annotation. *British Journal of Haematology*, **51**, 1982, 507–509.

Dickersin, G.R., Kline, I.W., and Scully, R.E. Small cell carcinoma of the ovary with hypercalcemia: A report of eleven cases. *Cancer*, **49**(1), 1982, 188–197.

Doogan, R.A. Hypercalcemia of malignancy. *Cancer Nursing.* **4**(4), 1981, 299–304.

Edsall, R.L. Probing the causes of hypercalcemia. *Patient Care*, **16**(2), 1982, 41–51.

Edsall, R.L. When you suspect hypercalcemia. *Patient Care*, **16**(2), 1982, 14–37.

Fields, A.L.A., Josse, R.G., and Bergsagel, D.E. Metabolic emergencies. In V.T. DeVita, et al. (eds.), *Cancer: Principles and practice of oncology*. Philadelphia: J. B. Lippincott Co., 1982.

Gordon, M. *Manual of nursing diagnosis*. New York: McGraw-Hill, 1982.

Guthrie, H.A. *Introductory nutrition* (4th ed.). St. Louis: C. V. Mosby, 1979.

Hayward, M.L., et al. Hypercalcemia complicating small-cell carcinoma. *Cancer*, **48**, 1981, 1643–1646.

Lukert, B.P. Hypercalcemia. *Critical Care Quarterly*, Aspen Systems Corporation, 1980, 11–18.

Megliola, B. Multiple myeloma. *Cancer Nursing*, **3**(3), 1980, 209–218.

Mundy, G.R., and Martin, T.J. The hypercalcemia of malignancy: Pathogenesis and management. *Metabolism*, **31**(12), 1982, 1247–1277.

Portlock, C.S., and Goffinet, D.R. *Manual of clinical problems in oncology*, Boston: Little, Brown, 1981, chap. 10.

Quinlan, M. Solving the mysteries of calcium imbalance: An action guide. *RN*, **45**(1), 1982, 50–54, 100.

Sneid, D. Hypercalcemia. *Topics in Emergency Medicine*, **5**(2), 1983, 8–17.

Stewart, A.F., et al. Hypercalcemia associated with gynecologic malignancies. *Cancer*, **49**(11), 1982, 2389–2394.

Zeluff, G.W., Suki, N.N., and Jackson, D. Hypercalcemia—Etiology, manifestations, and management. *Heart and Lung*, **9**(1), 1980, 146–151.

2. Hypophosphatemia

DEFINITION AND CAUSATIVE FACTORS

Hypophosphatemia occurs in the client with cancer when the serum concentration is less than 3.0 mg/dl; the normal level is 3.0 to 4.5 mg/dl. Hypophosphatemia is commonly associated with hypercalcemia, hypokalemia, hypomagnesemia, respiratory alkalosis, and ketoacidosis. It is frequently induced by aggressive hyperalimentation and parenteral nutrition therapy (TPN) because of an accelerated influx of phosphorus during carbohydrate metabolism. Normally, phosphorus (or phosphate) is regulated in the body by the same feedback mechanisms that regulate calcium (Chapter 1), primarily by the parathyroid hormone (PTH), secreted by the parathyroid, and vitamin D. PTH regulates the rate of reabsorption by the kidneys, and vitamin D determines the rate of absorption by the GI tract. Seventy percent of dietary phosphorus is absorbed by the GI tract, 90% becomes insoluble calcium phosphate, and 10% is located within the cell. Phosphorus and calcium are essential in the calcification of bones and teeth, and phosphorus is involved in almost all biological reactions requiring energy in the form of adenosine triphosphate (ATP), and is required in the active forms of vitamins, enzymes, DNA and RNA. Phosphorus also functions as a buffer to maintain an acid–base balance for the transport of nutrients into the cell, and in the structure of cells.

With a severe depletion of phosphorus the body is deprived of ATP, causing many incompleted biologic reactions resulting in red blood cell hemolysis, cardiomyopathy (Chapter 16), metabolic encephalopathy, and infection. In an attempt to compensate the deficiency, demineralization of bone can occur.

Corresponding cancers include multiple myeloma, leukemia, and other tumors that contain and secrete PTH. Malabsorption, bacterial sepsis, ketoacidosis, phosphate binding antacids (Amphogel), hyperparathyroidism, diuretics, corticosteroids, alcoholism, and thrombocytopenia are other additional causes.

ASSESSMENT DATA

- Serum phosphate levels less than 3.0 mg/dl
- Long-term parenteral nutrition or hyperalimentation
- Fatigue and weakness
- Anorexia
- Irritability
- Paresthesia
- Seizures

- Coma
- Respiratory alkalosis
- Thrombocytopenia
- Hypercalcemia
- Hypokalemia
- Hypomagnesemia
- Pathologic fractures
- Ketoacidosis

NURSING DIAGNOSES

Decreased activity tolerance, related to fatigue, weakness, and paresthesia resulting from a decreased serum phosphorous concentration.

Associated Nursing Diagnoses

1. Potential for physical injury, related to demineralization of bones and possible pathologic fractures, resulting from a phosphorus deficit.
2. Alteration in nutrition, more than body requirements, related to hyperalimentation and TPN, resulting in hypophosphatemia.
3. Impaired thought processes, related to irritability, seizures, and coma, resulting from hypophosphatemia.
4. Alteration in cardiac output, decreased, related to cardiomyopathy, resulting from decreased serum phosphorus levels.

RATIONALE

Interference with high energy phosphate bonding causes cellular energy depletion.

Organic matrix of bone is composed principally of phosphate and calcium.

Accelerated influx of phosphorus during carbohydrate metabolism.

Alteration in the shape and size of red blood cells interferes with adequate oxygen exchange.

Loss of high energy PO_4 bonds reduces the heart's ability to contract.

NURSING INTERVENTIONS

Monitoring–Independent

1. Assess client's tolerance for activity and subjective indications of weakness and fatigue with each contact.
2. Assess LOC q 4 to 8 hr and record changes in awareness, orientation, and behavior.
3. Assess client for anorexia at mealtime and record amount of food eaten.
4. Accurate I and O and calculate I/O ratio for fluid balance q 8 and 24 hr.
5. Assess client for complaints of bone pain q 4 to 8 hr.
6. BP, heart rate, and respirations q 2 hr.
7. Auscultate heart sounds in 4 valvular sites q 8 hr and record onset of extra heart sounds.
8. Palpate peripheral pulses for bilateral quality q 8 hr.
9. Assess neck vein distention q 8 hr and record in cm.
10. Inspect all dependent areas for edema q 8 hr.
11. Assess skin color, temperature, moisture, and discolorations q 4 to 8 hr.
12. Hemocult all stools and emesis with platelet count less than 50,000 cu mm.
13. Auscultate breath sounds in all lung fields q 8 hr and record onset of adventitious sounds.
14. Temperature q 4 hr.
15. Assess cardiac rhythm strip for abnormal changes in rhythm q 2 to 4 hr for decreased potassium level (prominent U wave, premature contractions, and tachyarrhythmias), and for increased calcium level (prolonged P-R interval and bradycardia).
16. Auscultate bowel sounds in 4 quadrants q 8 hr and record changes in pitch and frequency.
17. Weigh q AM before breakfast and record.

Monitoring–Interdependent

1. Assess results of laboratory data when available and compare to previous and normal values:
    Serum Phosphorus: 3.0 to 4.5 mg/dl
    Serum Sodium: 135 to 145 mEq/L
    Serum Potassium: 3.5 to 5.0 mEq/L
    Serum Chloride: 100 to 106 mEq/L
    Serum Calcium: 8.5 to 10.5 mg/dl
    Serum Magnesium: 1.5 to 2.0 mEq/L

Platelets: 130,000 to 370,000 mm^3

CBC   Hemoglobin: 13.0 to 18.0 g/dl males
                12.0 to 16.0 g/dl females
        Hematocrit: 45 to 52% males
                37 to 48% females
        RBC: 4.6 to 6.2 $\times$ 10^6/mm^3 males
                4.2 to 5.4 $\times$ 10^6/mm^3 females
        MCH: 27 to 32 pg
        MCHC: 32 to 36%
        MCV: 80 to 94 cu microns
        WBC: 4,500 to 11,500/mm^3

ABGs pH: 7.35 to 7.45
        Po_2: 75 to 100 torr
        Pco_2: 35 to 45 torr
        HCO_3: 24 to 30 mEq/L
        O_2 Saturation: 95 to 100%
        BE: $\pm$2 mEq/L
        CO_2 Content: 24 to 30 mEq/L

2. Assess client for hyperphosphatemia after initiation of phosphorus replacement therapy:
     Serum phosphorus levels greater than 4.5 mg/dl
     Sudden hypocalcemia from combining with excessive phosphorus
     Acute renal failure from deposition of calcium phosphate in renal parenchyma or collecting tubules

3. Assess TPN site for redness, pain, swelling q 8 hr.

Change-Independent

1. Maintain bedrest and minimize activity with serum phosphorus levels less than 3.0 mg/dl.

2. Institute all safety measures by elevating side rails, padding if client is restless or in danger of seizuring, and placing call light and personal articles within easy reach.

3. Reorient to time, place, and reason for hospitalization with each contact if client is confused or disoriented.

4. Offer fluids to 120 ml q 1 hr alternating with fat free milk and citrus juices (sources of phosphorus and potassium). Milk may be contraindicated if hypercalcemia present.

5. Position for maximum comfort and protection of fragile bones.

6. Mouth care after meals and bedtime using soft toothbrush and mouthwash. Once a day, clean teeth with a mixture of H_2O_2 and baking soda to neutralize oral acid and remove plaque.

7. Passive ROME to all major joints while on bedrest q 4 hr.

8. Turn, cough, deep breathe q 2 hr while on bedrest.

9. Back care q 4 hr while on bedrest and massage all bony prominences with lotion.

10. Institute gradual increase in activity when client can tolerate it or when prescribed by physician.

11. O_2 at 2 L/min by nasal cannula if SOB occurs.

12. Assist client to perform ADLs and maintain judicious independence and control over self and environment within physical limitations.

13. Explain condition and progress to client and family with each contact. Assist them to ask questions and express concerns of the present and the future.

14. Include family members in plan of care and allow them to participate, if mutually beneficial.

Change–Interdependent

1. Notify physician if:
   Serum phosphorus levels less than 3.0 mg/dl or greater than 4.5 mg/dl during or after replacement therapy
   Serum calcium levels greater than 10.5 mg/dl or less than 8.5 mg/dl during or after replacement therapy
   Serum potassium levels less than 3.5 mEq/L
   Serum magnesium levels less than 1.5 mEq/L
   Blood pH greater than 7.45 or less than 7.35
   Client develops seizures or becomes comatose
   Life-threatening arrhythmias develop
   Platelet count less than 50,000 cu mm
   Sudden onset of bone pain occurs
   Urinary output less than 30 ml/hr or 1500 ml less than intake/24 hr
   Positive cultures indicating bacterial sepsis

2. Anticipate physician to prescribe:
   15 to 30 ml $Na_2 HPO_4$ 3 to 4 times a day (Neutra-Phos) po (preferred)
   2.5 mg/kg body weight IV sodium or potassium phosphate if client not experiencing hypercalcemia, renal failure, tissue injury
   Potassium and magnesium supplementation may also be necessary because hypokalemia and hypomagnesemia are often associated with hypophosphatemia
   Discontinuation of Amphogel or other phosphorus binders
   Correction of ketoacidosis or respiratory alkalosis
   Intervention for thrombocytopenia (Chapter 10)

BIBLIOGRAPHY

Aderka, D., et al. Life-threatening hypophosphatemia in a patient with acute myelogenous leukemia. *Acta Haematology,* **64** (2), 1980, 117.

Corbett, J.V. *Laboratory Tests in Nursing Practice.* Norwalk, Connecticut, Appleton-Century-Crofts, 1982.

Gordon, M. *Manual of Nursing Diagnosis.* New York, McGraw-Hill, 1982.

Guthrie, H.A. *Introductory Nutrition.* (4th ed.). St. Louis, C. V. Mosby, 1979.

Horton, J., and Hill, G.J. *Clinical Oncology.* Philadelphia, W. B. Saunders, 1977.

Kliger, A.S., and Lovett, D.H. Electrolyte abnormalities in cancer patients. In J. Yarbro and R. Bornstein (eds.), *Oncologic Emergencies.* New York, Grune and Stratton, 1981.

Shoenfeld, Y., et al. Hypophosphatemia as diagnostic aid in sepsis. *New York State Journal of Medicine,* No. 2, February, 1982, pp. 163–165.

3. Hyponatremia

DEFINITION AND CAUSATIVE FACTORS

Hyponatremia unrelated to secretion of inappropriate ADH (SIADH) is characterized by serum sodium levels of 130 mEq/L or less and extracellular and intracellular body fluid depletion. Usually, symptoms do not occur until the serum sodium level reaches 120 mEq/L or less, and neurologic manifestations will occur at 110 mEq/L. Indications of fluid volume deficit vary according to a variety of factors, but a systolic blood pressure of 90 torr or less is usually cause for intervention. The causes of hyponatremia and fluid volume deficit in the client with cancer are related to liver, thyroid, and adrenal insufficiencies, kidney failure, and CHF. Intracranial neoplasms can cause a condition known as cerebral salt wasting in which the kidney is unable to conserve sodium due to a postulated natriuretic factor released by the brain or an alteration in neural innervation to the kidney. Aggressive diuretic therapy and high dose cyclophosphamide therapy can also produce serious hyponatremia and fluid volume deficit.

Dilutional hyponatremia can occur when the serum sodium concentration is within normal limits, but the fluid volume is expanded resulting in hyponatremic measurements. It is caused by excessive water intake, hypothyroidism, and adrenal insufficiency and is determined by urine sodium levels which equal the sodium intake. True hyponatremia with normovolemia occurs with SIADH, poor salt intake, or irrigating NG tubes with water washing out the gastric sodium. False or pseudohyponatremia occurs with hyperlipidemia, hyperproteinemia associated with multiple myeloma, hyperglycemia, and mannitol administration.

If the sodium loss is caused by nonrenal etiology, the urine sodium level is less than 10 mEq/L; renal insufficiency results in urine sodium levels greater than 50 mEq/L.

Corresponding cancers include lung, pancreas, duodenum, larynx, leukemia, brain, esophagus, colon, ovary, prostate, bronchus, Hodgkin, lymphosarcoma, and multiple myeloma. Diuretics, chlorpropamide, narcotics, barbiturates, clofibrate, isoproterenol, tolbutamide, CHF, and adrenal and renal insufficiency are additional factors. High dose cyclophosphamide chemotherapy and a decrease in the peripheral blast cell count due to daunorubicin or cytosine chemotherapy are subsequent causative factors to clients with cancer.

ASSESSMENT DATA

- Serum sodium level less than 130 mEq/L *plus*
- Urine sodium levels less than 20 mEq/L or greater than 50 mEq/L
- Hypokalemia or hyperkalemia
- Serum hypoosmolality
- Thirst
- Headache
- Postural hypotension
- Anorexia
- Nausea and vomiting
- Muscle cramps
- Diarrhea
- Cold, clammy skin with poor turgor

- Tachycardia
- Hypercalcemia
- Edema or ascites with dilutional hyponatremia
- With serum sodium levels 110 mEq/L or less:
  Restlessness
  Confusion
  Muscle twitching
  Seizures
  Coma
- With chronic hyponatremia:
  Hemiparesis
  Ataxia
  Babinski reflex

NURSING DIAGNOSES

Alteration in fluid volume, deficit, related to a decreased concentration of serum sodium resulting in extracellular fluid depletion.

Associated Nursing Diagnoses

1. Alteration in fluid volume, excess, related to dilutional hyponatremia, resulting in fluid volume excess and edema.

RATIONALE

Excessive excretion of body sodium is caused by both renal and nonrenal etiologies or the dilutional body phenomenon. Diminished extracellular fluid volume, blood volume; and arterial pressure results.

Water retention is proportionally greater than sodium retention; hence, hypotonic hyponatremia. Occurs in CHF, acute renal failure, cirrhosis, or hypoproteinemia.

2. Alteration in sensory perception, related to a decrease in
   LOC resulting from serum
   sodium levels less than 110
   mEq/L.

Sodium gradient theory states that
sodium must be present in order
for glucose to be transported
into cells; hence, essential for
neurologic functioning.

3. Potential for physical injury,
   related to ataxia and hemiparesis, resulting from chronic
   hyponatremia.

Sodium gradient theory. Sodium is
essential for muscular
functioning.

NURSING INTERVENTIONS

Monitoring–Independent

1. Accurate I and O and calculate I/O ratio for fluid balance q 8 and 24 hr.
2. Assess skin color, temperature, moisture, and turgor q 8 hr.
3. Weight q AM before breakfast and compare to previous weight.
4. Urine specific gravity q 4 to 8 hr.
5. Assess client for nausea and vomiting with each contact and for anorexia at mealtime.
6. Oral temperature q 4 hr.
7. Assess LOC q 4 to 8 hr and record changes in awareness, orientation, and
   behavior.
8. BP, heart rate, and respirations q 2 to 4 hr.
9. Assess client for weakness and ataxia while ambulating.
10. Assess all dependent areas for edema q 8 hr.
11. Auscultate heart sounds in 4 valvular sites q 8 hr and record onset of
    gallop.
12. Palpate peripheral pulses for bilateral quality q 8 hr.
13. Auscultate breath sounds in all lung fields q 8 hr and record onset of
    adventitious sounds.
14. Assess IV site for redness, pain, swelling q 4 to 8 hr.

Monitoring–Interdependent

1. Assess laboratory data when available and compare to previous and
   normal values.
   Serum Sodium: 135 to 145 mEq/L
   Serum Potassium: 3.5 to 5.0 mEq/L

Serum Chloride: 100 to 106 mEq/L
Serum Calcium: 8.5 to 10.5 mg/dl
Serum Osmolality: 286 to 294 mOsm/kg
BUN: 8 to 25 mg/dl
Creatinine: 0.6 to 1.5 mg/dl
Urine Osmolality: 50 to 1200 mOsm/kg/H_2O (average: 200 to 800)
Urine Sodium: 40 to 220 mEq/L/24 hr
Urine Potassium: 25 to 120 mEq/L/24 hr

2. Assess client for fluid volume overload if physician prescribes IV normal saline and/or volume expanders:
   BP greater than 40 torr systolic from baseline (approximate)
   Polyuria
   Onset of edema, rales, rhonchi, bounding apical pulse
3. Assess client for packed RBC transfusion reaction if appropriate:
   Fever, chills
   Tachypnea, wheezing
   Lumbar pain
   Nausea
   Dyspnea, rales
   Chest pain
   Hives

Change–Independent

1. Maintain bedrest with minimized activity with serum sodium level less than 120 mEq/L.
2. Turn, cough, deep breathe q 2 hr while on bedrest.
3. Bathe without soap using commercially prepared bath emollient BID.
4. Apply ice collar to neck with onset of nausea.
5. Back care and massage all bony prominences with lotion q 4 hr.
6. Mouth care using soft toothbrush and oral antiseptic q 4 hr or after meals. Once a day, clean teeth with mixture of H_2O_2 and baking soda to neutralize oral acid and remove plaque.
7. Passive ROME to all major joints q 4 hr while on bedrest.
8. Institute all safety measures. Keep side rails up and pad if client is restless or disoriented, place call light and personal articles within easy reach, and ambulate with assistance.
9. Before all procedures, explain purpose and technique in understandable terms.
10. Reorient to time, place, and reason for hospitalization if client is confused or disoriented.

11. Assist client to perform ADLs and maintain judicious independence over self and environment within physical limitations.
12. Explain condition and progress to client and family with each contact. Assist to ask questions and express concerns to the present and the future.
13. Include family members in plan of care and allow them to participate if mutually beneficial.

Change–Interdependent

1. Notify physician if:
   Serum Sodium less than 120 mEq/L
   Serum Potassium less than 3.5 mEq/L
   Serum Calcium greater than 10.5 mg/dl
   Serum Osmolality less than 280 mOsm/kg
   Changes in LOC
   Weight gain or loss of 1 to 2 kg/day
   Systolic BP less than 90 torr or greater than 160 torr
   Transfusion reaction occurs
2. Discontinue blood transfusion if rales, fever, lumbar or chest pain, or dyspnea occurs.
3. Anticipate physician to prescribe:
   Change in chemotherapy orders
   IV normal saline with fluid volume deficit to increase volume
   Colloidal volume expanders with fluid volume deficit
   Fluid restriction with dilutional hyponatremia
   Packed RBCs to expand volume
   Potassium added to IV fluids to correct hypokalemia
   Antiemetic and antidiarrheal medications
4. Medicate appropriately for nausea, vomiting, diarrhea, and assess effect in 30 min.

BIBLIOGRAPHY

Ashraf, N., Locksley, R., and Arieff, A.I. Thiazide-induced hyponatremia associated with death or neurologic damage in outpatients. *The American Journal of Medicine,* **70,** 1981, 1163–1174.
Barber, J.M., and Budassi, S.A. *Manual of Emergency Care—Practices and Procedures.* St. Louis, C.V. Mosby, 1979.
Boh, D.M., and Van Son, A.R. The water-load test. *American Journal of Nursing,* **82**(1), 1982, 112–113.
Corbett, J.V. *Laboratory Tests in Nursing Practice.* Norwalk, Connecticut, Appleton-Century-Crofts, 1982.

Goldberg, M. Hyponatremia. *Medical Clinics of North America*, 65(2), 1981, 251–269.

Gordon, M. *Manual of Nursing Diagnosis*. New York: McGraw-Hill, 1982.

Gray, S. Hyponatremia and its relationship to clients with cancer. Presented at the *Second Oncology Nursing Seminar, Clemson University,* College of Nursing, Clemson, South Carolina, May 1982.

Hamburger, S., and Rush, D. Syndrome of inappropriate secretion of antidiuretic hormone. *Critical Care Quarterly,* Aspen Systems Corporation, 1980, 119–129.

Kee, J.L. *Laboratory and Diagnostic Tests with Nursing Implications.* Norwalk, Connecticut, Appleton-Century-Crofts, 1983.

Nelson, P.B., Seif, S.M., Maroon, J.C., and Robinson, A.G. Hyponatremia in intracranial disease: Perhaps not the syndrome of inappropriate secretion of antidiuretic hormone (SIADH). *Journal of Neurosurgery,* 55 1981, 938–941.

Thomas, A.G. Disorders of sodium metabolism. In S. Hamburger (ed.), *Topics in Emergency medicine* (vol. 5, no. 2). Aspen Systems Corporation, July 1983, pp. 46–50.

Trump, D.L. Serious hyponatremia in patients with cancer: Management with demeclocycline. *Cancer,* 47, 1981, 2908–2912.

4. Hypokalemia

DEFINITION AND CAUSATIVE FACTORS

Hypokalemia is defined as a serum potassium concentration of 3.0 mEq/L or less; the normal value is between 3.5 tp 5.0 mEq/L. Normally, potassium balance is maintained in the body by several regulatory mechanisms: dietary intake, renal conservation or elimination, aldosterone production, and GI tract excretion. The usual daily dietary intake is approximately 40 to 100 mEq (1500 to 4000 mg). Ninety-eight percent of potassium is contained within the cell and 2% in extracellular fluid. Ninety percent of dietary potassium is excreted by the kidneys and 10% by the GI tract. Aldosterone is hypokalemic hormone; it promotes cellular uptake of potassium and renal excretion. The distal convoluted tubule of the nephron has the ability to actively conserve or excrete potassium depending on the body's state of deficit or excess. Potassium functions to control intracellular osmotic pressure, neuromuscular activity, muscle excitability, acid–base balance, and glucose transport.

Hypokalemia has four principal causes: intercellular shift, excess loss by the kidney, excess loss by the GI tract, or insufficient dietary intake. Potassium, like many other minerals, can be stored by the body, but its supply can be easily depleted. Potassium loss by the GI tract occurs with diarrhea, vomiting, or NG tube continuous suctioning. Only 5 to 10 mEq of potassium is located in the stomach, but with severe vomiting or suctioning, hydrogen is removed resulting in alkalosis and hypokalemia as the body attempts to compensate by exchanging extracelluar potassium for intracellular hydrogen. The lower GI tract has much higher amounts of potassium, and severe diarrhea can cause rapid depletion. The client with cancer who is anorexic, vomiting, or NPO, suffers a deficient dietary intake. Cancers causing excessive diarrhea include gastrin–producing tumors of the non-β islet pancreatic cells (Zollinger–Ellison syndrome); pancreatic tumors that elaborate vasoactive intestinal polypeptides, prostaglandins, and other hormones (pancreatic cholera syndrome); medullary carcinoma of the thyroid; carcinoid intestinal tumors that cause intestinal hypermotility; and villinous carcinoma of the colon that can cause stool volumes up to 1500 to 3500 ml/day.

Excessive loss of potassium through urinary excretion is caused by diuretics, hypercalcemia, hypomagnesemia, and several antibiotics. Cancers causing kaluresis are adrenal adenoma producing hyperaldosteronism, adrenal hyperplasia tumors resulting in excess corticosteriods (Cushing syndrome), cancer cells that produce ACTH independently (ectopic ACTH syndrome), and renin–secreting intrarenal tumors. Hodgkin disease, multiple myeloma, and acute blast crisis are associated with renal tubular necrosis and kaluresis. Myelomonocytic leukemia causes an increase in serum lysozyme which interferes with renal tubular function resulting in kaluresis. Serum sodium excess or deficit may be a concurrent problem.

Ileostomy, colostomy, fistulas, diuretic phase of renal failure, ulcerative colitis, antibiotics carbenicillin, ticarcillin, amphoteric B, gentamycin administration, and nephrotoxicity caused by chemotherapy and radiation therapy are additional causes of hypokalemia.

ASSESSMENT DATA

- Serum potassium levels less than 3.0 mEq/L
- EKG changes
  Prominent U wave
  T wave inversion
  Depressed (sagging ST segment)
  TU fusion
  Premature contractions
  Atrial tachycardia
  Atrial flutter
- Cardiac arrhythmias—PACs PVCs, tachycardia, atrial flutter, ventricular fibrillation, or asystole
- Nausea and vomiting
- Anorexia
- Distended abdomen
- Paralytic ileus
- Weakness
- Fatigue
- Hypoactive deep tendon reflexes
- Cramps
- Paresthesia
- Digitalis toxicity
- Glucose intolerance (hyperglycemia)
- Alkalosis
- Hypomagnesemia
- Hypercalcemia
- SOB
- Respiratory arrest

NURSING DIAGNOSES	RATIONALE
Fluid volume deficit, related to loss of fluid from excessive excretion by	*Stomach and/or GI tract evacuation result in overt loss of fluid*

NURSING DIAGNOSES

RATIONALE

diarrhea or diuresis, resulting in hypokalemia.

volume and dietary potassium. Diuresis enhances loss of potassium via kidney excretion disallowing the regulatory mechanism of renal conservation.

Associated Nursing Diagnoses

1. Alterations in nutrition, less than body requirements, related to excessive diarrhea, nausea, anorexia, or vomiting, resulting in hypokalemia and undernutrition.

Two regulatory mechanisms are impeded: dietary intake and GI tract excretion.

2. Potential for physical injury, related to weakness, fatigue, and paresthesia, resulting from hypokalemia.

Hyperpolarization of nerve and muscle fiber membranes prevents transmission of action potentials.

NURSING INTERVENTIONS

Monitoring–Independent

1. Assess cardiac rhythm strip for indications of hypokalemia (Fig. 4-1) (also, ventricular tachycardia and fibrillation).
2. Assess client for nausea with each contact and record amount and character of emesis.
3. Record amount of each diarrheal stool and describe color and consistency.
4. Accurate I and O and calculate I/O ratio for fluid balance q 8 and 24 hr.
5. BP, heart rate, and respirations q 2 hr with frequent episodes of vomiting and diarrhea.
6. Temperature q 4 hr.
7. Weigh q AM before breakfast and compare to previous measurements.
8. Assess client's tolerance for activity and subjective indications of weakness and fatigue q 4 to 8 hr.
9. Assess skin color, temperature, moisture, and turgor q 8 hr.

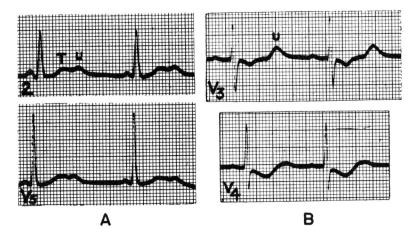

Figure 4-1. Hypokalemia. Tracings **A** and **B** are different patients. **A** shows early changes of hypokalemia with prominent U wave merging to form continuous undulating wave with T wave. **B** shows changes of advanced hypokalemia (1.8 mEq/L) in a patient with cirrhosis; note ST depression with very prominent U waves in V₃. Source: Marriott, H.J.L., 1977, with permission.

10. Assess urine sugar and acetone q 6 hr.

11. Assess LOC q 8 hr and record changes in awareness, orientation, and behavior.

12. Auscultate bowel sounds in 4 quadrants for character and frequency of sounds q 4 to 8 hr and onset of high pitched or absent sounds.

13. Auscultate heart sounds in 4 valvular sites q 8 hr and record onset of extra heart sounds.

14. Palpate peripheral pulses for bilateral quality q 8 hr.

15. Auscultate breath sounds in all lung fields q 8 hr and record onset of SOB or increased respiratory effort.

16. Assess for dependent edema q 8 hr.

Monitoring–Interdependent

1. Assess results of laboratory data when available and compare to previous and normal values.

    Serum Potassium: 3.5 to 5.0 mEq/L
    Serum Sodium: 135 to 145 mEq/L
    Serum Chloride: 100 to 106 mEq/L
    Serum Calcium: 8.5 to 10.5 mg/dl
    Serum Magnesium: 1.5 to 2.0 mEq/L

    ABGs pH: 7.35 to 7.45
            Po_2: 75 to 100 torr
            Pco_2: 35 to 45 torr
            HCO_3: 24 to 30 mEq/L
            CO_2 Content: 24 to 30 mEq/L
            BE: ± 2 mEq/L
            O_2 Saturation: 95 to 100%
    BUN: 8 to 25 mg/dl
    Creatinine: 0.6 to 1.5 mg/dl
    Digoxin Level: therapeutic range = 0.8 to 1.6 ng/ml
    Blood Sugar: 70 to 110 mg/dl

2. Assess IV site for redness, pain, swelling, and indications of phlebitis along vein tract proximal to IV site q 4 to 8 hr.
3. Assess client for hyperkalemia after initiation of potassium replacement therapy.

    Tall, peaked T waves on EKG
    Hyperactive deep tendon reflexes
    Nausea and vomiting
    Serum potassium levels greater than 5 mEq/L

Change–Independent

1. Maintain bedrest and minimize activity with serum potassium levels less than 3.0 mEq/L.
2. Offer fluids to 150 ml q 1 hr while awake with high potassium fluids— citrus fruit juice, milk, banana milk shakes, apple juice if tolerated or if active nausea or vomiting absent.
3. Perirectal skin care after each diarrheal stool using protective skin agent.
4. Apply ice collar to neck with onset of nausea.
5. Mouth care q 4 hr and after each vomiting episode and before meals using appropriate oral antiseptic that is refreshing without tasting too sweet. Once a day, clean teeth with a mixture of H_2O_2 and baking soda to neutralize oral acid and remove plaque.
6. Passive ROME to all major extremities while on bedrest q 4 hr.
7. Turn, cough, deep breathe q 2 hr while on bedrest.
8. Back care q 4 hr while on bedrest and massage all bony prominences with lotion.
9. Institute gradual increase in activity when client can tolerate it or when prescribed by physician.
10. O_2 at 2 L/min by nasal cannula if SOB occurs.
11. Institute all safety measures by elevating side rails and pad if client

restless or disoriented; place bed in low position, and place call light and personal articles within easy reach.

12. Assist client to perform ADLs and maintain judicious independence and control over self and environment within physical limitations.

13. Explain condition and progress to client and family with each contact. Assist them to ask questions and express concerns of the present and the future.

14. Include family members in plan of care and allow them to participate if mutually beneficial.

Change–Interdependent

1. Normal saline at KVO or as prescribed by physician.

2. Medicate appropriately as prescribed for vomiting, diarrhea, and arrhythmias and assess effect in 1 to 30 min.

3. Notify physician if:

Serum potassium less than 3.0 mEq/L or greater than 5.0 mEq/L during or after replacement therapy

Serum calcium greater than 11.0 mg/dl

Serum magnesium less than 1.5 mEq/L

Serum blood sugar greater than 250 mg/dl

Blood pH greater than 7.45

BUN greater than 25 mg/dl *and*

Creatinine greater than 1.5 mg/dl

EKG changes occur indicating arrhythmia or presence of U wave

High pitched or absent bowel sounds with abdominal distention

Digoxin level greater than 1.9 ng/ml

4. Anticipate physician to prescribe:

IV normal saline to restore volume

Potassium chloride supplements: amount and route depends on degree of hypokalemia. With a serum potassium level of 3.0 mEq/L, there is a 100 to 200 mEq deficit. For every 1 mEq/L decrease thereafter there is a 200 to 400 mEq deficit. IV concentration should not exceed 60 to 80 mEq/L of IV fluid and 30 to 40 ml/hr.

Antiemetic and antidiarrheal medications

Surgical removal of tumor contributing to hypokalemia

Magnesium supplementation may be required because hypomagnesemia is often associated with hypokalemia

Correction of metabolic alkalosis

Change in antibiotic therapy

Change in chemotherapy and/or radiation therapy

BIBLIOGRAPHY

Corbett, J.V. *Laboratory Tests in Nursing Practice.* Norwalk, Connecticut: Appleton-Century-Crofts, 1982.

Donovan, M.I., and Pierce, S.G. *Cancer Care Nursing.* New York: Appleton-Century-Crofts, 1976.

Fletcher, B. *Quick Reference to Critical Care Nursing.* Philadelphia: J. B. Lippincott, 1983.

Gordon, M. *Manual of Nursing Diagnosis.* New York: McGraw-Hill, 1982.

Guthrie, H.A. *Introductory Nutrition* (4th ed). St. Louis: C.V. Mosby, 1979.

Horton, J., and Hill, G.J. *Clinical Oncology.* Philadelphia: W.B. Saunders, 1977.

Issacs, M. Life threatening fluid and electrolyte abnormalities in patients with cancer. In A.D. Turnbull (ed.), *Current Problems in Cancer*, (vol. 4, no. 3.). Chicago, Year Book Medical Publishers, 1979, 10.

Kliger, A.S., and Lovett, D.H. Electrolyte abnormalities in cancer patients. In J. Yarbro and R. Bornstein (eds.), *Oncologic Emergencies.* New York: Grune and Stratton, 1981.

Kosmidis, P., Jamse, K.M. and Axelrod, A.R. Hypokalemia in leukemia. *Annals Internal Medicine*, **82**, 1975, 854–855.

Kunau, R.T., and Stein, J.H. Disorders of hypo- and hyperkalemia. *Clinical Nephrology*, **7**, 1977, 173.

Luckman, J., and Sorensen, K.C. *Medical-Surgical Nursing—A Psychophysiologic Approach* (2nd ed.). Philadelphia: W.B. Saunders, 1980.

Marriott, H.J.L. *Practical Electrocardiography* (6th ed.). Baltimore: Williams & Wilkins, 1977.

Menzel, L.K. Clinical problems of electrolyte balance. *Nursing Clinics of North America*, **15**(3), 1980, 559–576.

Mir, M.A., Brabin, B., Tang, O.T., et al. *Annals Internal Medicine*, **82**, 1975, 54–57.

Otrakji, J. Disorders of potassium metabolism. *Topics in Emergency Medicine*, **5**(2), 1983, 53–57.

Stolinsky, D.C. Emergencies in oncology—Current management. *The Western Journal of Medicine*, **129**(3), 1978, 169–176.

Ventricular arrhythmias from thiazide-induced hypokalemia. *Nurses Drug Alert*, **5**(8), August 1981, 79–80.

Wright, T.R., and Murray, M. Potassium problems: Which patient's in danger? *RN*, **45**(6), 1982, 57–61.

5. Hypomagnesemia

DEFINITION AND CAUSATIVE FACTORS

Hypomagnesemia is defined as a serum magnesium concentration less than 1.5 mEq/L; the normal value is between 1.5 and 2.0 mEq/L. Hypomagnesemia most often occurs in the client with cancer who is experiencing severe vomiting, diarrhea, malabsorption syndrome, malnutrition, ADH secreting tumors, and kidney disease, or is receiving cis-Platinum, nephrotoxic antibiotics, and long-term parenteral nutrition. The initial manifestation of hypomagnesemia is increased neuromuscular and nervous system hyperexcitability because magnesium suppresses the release of acetylcholine at neuromuscular junctions. Normally, magnesium is absorbed by the GI tract, becomes plasma protein bound, and about 50% combines with calcium and phosphorus in the bone, which becomes a storage site. Magnesium is primarily an intracellular mineral; only 1% is extracellular. It is regulated by the kidney with some influence from the parathyroid hormone.

Magnesium functions as an activator for the enzyme ATPase, which is necessary for the contraction of muscles and muscle repolarization, glucose utilization, and synthesis of fats and protein. Magnesium is also required in order to activate the regulation of calcium and potassium ions. In addition to neuromuscular excitability, a magnesium deficit can cause cardiac arrhythmias and metabolic encephalopathy. Magnesium deficits may be more common than potassium deficits.

Corresponding cancers include those treated with cis-Platinum (testicular, ovarian) and ADH secreting tumor, such as oat-cell carcinoma of the lung.

Increased thyroid, aldosterone, ADH, and parathyroid hormone activity, hydronephrosis, glomerulonephritis, pyelonephritis, renal tubular acidosis, diuretic therapy, bowel resection, ulcerative colitis, intestinal fistulae, alcoholism, and corticosteroids are other additional causes.

ASSESSMENT DATA

- Serum magnesium levels less than 1.5 mEq/L
- Prolonged parenteral nutrition without magnesium supplementation
- Muscle twitching
- Tremors
- Nystagmus
- Positive Chvostek sign
- Positive Trousseau sign
- Leg and foot cramps
- Hyperactive deep tendon reflexes
- Tetany

- Changes in LOC—restlessness, disorientation, and confusion
- Nausea and vomiting
- Convulsions
- Hypokalemia
- Hypocalcemia
- EKG changes:
    Prolonged PR interval
    Prolonged QT interval
    Broad, flat T waves
- Cardiac arrhythmias:
    Premature ventricular contractions
    Ventricular tachycardia
    Ventricular fibrillation

NURSING DIAGNOSES

Impaired physical mobility, related to hyperexcitability of neuro-muscular function, resulting from a magnesium deficit.

Associated Nursing Diagnoses

1. Potential for physical injury, related to possible tetany and convulsions, resulting from a magnesium deficit.
2. Alterations in cardiac output, decreased, related to ventricular arrythmias, which could result from a magnesium deficit.

RATIONALE

Increased release of acetylcholine at neuromuscular junctions.

Lack of activation of ATPase inhibits production of ATP causing delayed muscle contraction.

Inhibition of ATP production delays muscle contraction. The action of digitalis is also potentiated by hypomagnesemia.

NURSING INTERVENTIONS

Monitoring–Independent

1. Observe client for involuntary intention tremor (tremors occurring with fine or gross motor function) and muscle twitching with each contact.

2. Assess client q 8 hr for positive Trousseau sign by inflating blood pressure cuff for 1 to 5 min inducing carpal spasm and for positive Chvostek sign by tapping the facial nerve just below the temple inducing contraction of the nose, lip, and face indicating tetany.

3. Assess for nystagmus q 8 hr by asking client to follow an object (finger or pencil) to the far right, left, up and down, and observe for rapid movement of the eyeball.

4. Test deep tendon reflexes q 8 hr by tapping biceps, triceps, patellae, and Achilles tendon and record onset of exaggerated response.

5. Assess LOC q 4 to 8 hr and record changes in awareness, orientation, and behavior.

6. Accurate I and O and calculate I/O ratio for fluid balance q 8 and 24 hr.

7. Assess cardiac rhythm strip for abnormal changes in rhythm q 1 to 2 hr with decreasing magnesium levels and continuous monitoring with levels less than 1.0 mEq/L.

8. Assess client for unsteadiness of gait or weakness when ambulating.

9. BP, heart rate, respirations q 2 hr.

10. Temperature q 4 hr.

11. Assess skin color, temperature, and moisture q 8 hr.

12. Inspect all dependent areas for edema q 8 hr if client in renal failure.

13. Auscultate heart sounds in 4 valvular sites q 8 hr and record onset of extra heart sounds.

14. Auscultate breath sounds in all lung fields q 8 hr and record onset of adventitious sounds.

15. Auscultate bowel sounds in 4 quadrants q 8 hr and record changes in pitch and frequency of sound.

16. Weigh q AM before breakfast if client malnourished, receiving TPN, or in renal failure.

17. Document anthropometric measurements q 5 days.

Monitoring-Interdependent

1. Assess results of laboratory data when available and compare to previous and normal values.
   Serum Magnesium: 1.5 to 2.0 mEq/L
   Serum Sodium: 135 to 145 mEq/L
   Serum Potassium: 3.5 to 5.0 mEq/L
   Serum Chloride: 100 to 106 mEq/L
   Serum Calcium: 8.5 to 10.5 mg/dl
   BUN: 8 to 25 mg/dl
   Creatinine: 0.6 to 1.5 mg/dl

2. Assess client for hypermagnesemia after initiation of magnesium replacement therapy.

    Serum magnesium levels greater than 2.0 mEq/L

    Hypotension from vasodilatation

    Facial flushing from peripheral vasodilatation

    Cardiac or respiratory arrest from heart block, bradycardia and muscle paralysis

3. Assess IV site or TPN site for redness, swelling, and pain q 8 hr.

4. Assess results of anthropometric measurements when available and compare to table of standard values.

Change–Independent

1. Maintain bedrest and minimize activity with serum magnesium levels less than 1.5 mEq/L.

2. Institute all safety measures by elevating side rails and pad if client restless or exhibiting excessive involuntary body movement, or in danger of convulsing.

3. Reorient to time, place, and reason for hospitalization with each contact if client confused and disoriented.

4. Apply ice collar to neck with onset of nausea.

5. Peri-rectal skin care after each diarrheal stool using protective skin agent.

6. Mouth care q 4 hr and after each vomiting episode and before meals using appropriate oral antiseptic that is refreshing without tasting too sweet. Once a day, clean teeth with a mixture of H_2O_2 and baking soda to neutralize oral acid and remove plaque.

7. Passive ROME to all major joints while on bedrest q 4 hr.

8. Turn, cough, deep breathe q 2 hr while on bedrest.

9. Back care q 4 hr while on bedrest and massage all bony prominences with lotion.

10. Institute gradual increase in activity when client can tolerate it or when prescribed by physician.

11. O_2 at 2 L/min by nasal cannula if SOB occurs.

12. Assist client to perform ADLs and maintain judicious independence and control over self and environment within physical limitations.

13. Explain condition and progress to client and family with each contact. Assist them to ask questions and express concerns of the present and the future.

14. Include family members in plan of care and allow them to participate if mutually beneficial.

Change–Interdependent

1. D5W at KVO or as prescribed by physician.
2. Medicate appropriately for nausea, vomiting, or cardiac arrhythmias as prescribed and assess effect in 1 to 30 min.
3. Notify physician if:

> Serum magnesium levels less than 1.5 mEq/L or greater than 2.0 mEq/L during or after replacement therapy
> Serum calcium levels less than 8.5 mg/dl
> Serum potassium levels less than 3.5 mEq/L
> EKG changes or arrhythmias occur
> Convulsions or tetany occur
> Hypotension, bradycardia, decreased respirations, or urinary output less than 30 ml/hr after magnesium replacement instituted

4. Anticipate physician to prescribe:
Magnesium sulfate added to IV or TPN solution
> 2 mEq/kg body weight *or*
> 8 to 16 mEq IM *or*
> 0.25 to 0.5 mEq/kg body weight po
> IV or IM preferred since po magnesium sulfate causes diarrhea

Potassium and calcium supplements may also be necessary because hypokalemia and hypocalcemia are often associated with hypomagnesemia.

BIBLIOGRAPHY

Boyd, J.C., Bruns, D.E., and Wills, M.R. Frequency of hypomagnesemia in hypokalemia states. *Clinical Chemistry*, 29(1), 1983, 178–179.
Corbett, J.V. *Laboratory Tests in Nursing Practice*. Norwalk, Connecticut: Appleton-Century-Crofts, 1982.
Felver, L. Understanding the electrolyte maze. *American Journal of Nursing*, 80(9), 1980, 1591–1595.
Gordon, M. *Manual of Nursing Diagnosis*. New York: McGraw-Hill, 1982.
Guthrie, H.A. *Introductory Nutrition* (4th ed.). St. Louis: C.V. Mosby, 1979.
Horton, J., and Hill, G.J. *Clinical Oncology*. Philadelphia: W.B. Saunders, 1977.
Kliger, A.S., and Lovett, D.H. *Electrolyte abnormalities in cancer patients*. In J. Yarbro and R. Bornstein (eds.), *Oncologic Emergencies*. New York: Grune and Stratton, 1981.
Luckman, J., and Sorensen, K.C. *Medical-Surgical Nursing—A Psychophysiologic Approach* (2nd ed.). Philadelphia: W.B. Saunders, 1980.
Quinlan, M. Would you recognize this dangerous electrolyte imbalance? *RN*, 46(3), 1983, 51–55.

6. Hyperkalemia

DEFINITION AND CAUSATIVE FACTORS

Hyperkalemia is defined as a serum potassium concentration of 5.5 mEq/L or greater; the normal value is between 3.5 to 5.0 mEq/L. Normally, potassium balance is maintained in the body by several regulatory mechanisms: dietary intake, renal conservation or elimination, aldosterone production, and GI tract excretion. The usual daily dietary intake is approximately 40 to 100 mEq (1500 to 4000 mg). Ninety-eight percent of potassium is contained within the cell and 2% in extracellular fluid. Ninety percent of dietary potassium is excreted by the kidneys and 10% by the GI tract. Aldosterone regulates potassium levels by promoting cellular uptake and renal excretion. The distal convoluted tubule of the nephron has the ability to actively conserve or excrete potassium in states of deficit or excess. Potassium functions to control intracellular osmotic pressure, neuromuscular activity, muscle excitability, acid–base balance, and glucose transport.

Hyperkalemia has three principle causes: intracellular–extracellular redistribution, total body excess, and renal retention. The most common condition involving redistribution is respiratory or metabolic acidosis in which a compensatory shift of intracellular potassium for extracellular hydrogen occurs. Certain malignant cells produce high levels of lactic acid (acute lymphocytic leukemia, lymphosarcoma, Hodgkin disease, Burkitt lymphoma), and with liver metastasis, lactic acid cannot be sufficiently metabolized resulting in lactic acidosis. Total body excess occurs in the client with cancer because of toxic cell lysis in which massive amounts of potassium and other substances are released from destroyed malignant cells. If kidney function is normal, excess potassium excretion prevents sustained hyperkalemia. Red blood cell lysis is another cause of total body potassium excess. Renal retention of potassium is caused by renal failure and hypoaldosteronism (Addison disease). Serum sodium excess or deficit may be a concurrent electrolyte abnormality.

False or pseudohyperkalemia may occur in clients with high platelet and/or WBC counts of myeloproliferative diseases.

Corresponding cancers include acute leukemia, lymphosarcoma, Hodgkin disease, Burkitt lymphoma, oat cell carcinoma, and metastatic replacement of liver tissue. Rapid lysis of WBCs due to chemotherapy, renal failure, acidosis, renal obstruction, Addison disease (adrenal atrophy), and Dyrenium (triamterene) are additional causes.

ASSESSMENT DATA

- Serum potassium levels greater than 5.5 mEq/L
- EKG changes
  Tall, thin T waves
  Prolonged PR interval
  Depressed ST segment
  Wide QRS
  Absent P waves with severe potassium deficit
- Arrhythmias—A-V block, bradycardia, atrial standstill, ventricular fibrillation, and cardiac arrest
- Acidosis
- Hyperuricemia
- Hypocalcemia
- Hyperphosphatemia
- Muscle weakness
- Cramps in skeletal muscles

- Hyperactive reflexes
- Paresthesia
- Abdominal cramps
- Nausea
- Diarrhea
- Paralytic ileus
- Renal failure
  Hypertension
  Anemia
  Weight gain
  Edema
  Pulmonary congestion
  Increased BUN and creatinine
  Oliguria, anuria, polyuria
  Hypernatremia
  Decreased creatinine clearance

NURSING DIAGNOSES

Fluid volume excess related to fluid retention that results when the serum potassium levels increase sufficiently to require dilution.

RATIONALE

Toxic cell lysis due to chemotherapy and/or a buildup of lactic acid released by certain cancer cells causes a shift in potassium from ICF to ECF. (If blood transfusion is required, fresh blood must be used for clients who have potassium intoxication. Stored blood tends to release potassium.)

Associated Nursing Diagnoses

1. Potential for physical injury related to paresthesias and muscle weakness, resulting from hyperkalemia.

   Potassium decreases membrane potential producing overstimulation of nerve impulses and eventual muscle weakness.

2. Alterations in nutrition, less than body requirements, related to nausea, vomiting, anorexia, and possible paralytic ileus, resulting from hyperkalemia.

   Burning of fat for energy produces ketones, and as proteins are burned, potassium is liberated.

3. Altered urinary elimination, decreased, related to the inability of the kidney to excrete fluid and electrolytes, resulting in hyperkalemia and fluid retention.

   Impaired renal function causes retention of potassium and fluid.

4. Altered cardiac output, decreased, related to possible life-threatening cardiac arrhythmias, resulting from hyperkalemia.

   Depolarization of the membranes of cardiac muscle causes weakness in heart muscle contraction and eventual arrhythmias.

NURSING INTERVENTIONS

Monitoring–Independent

1. Assess cardiac rhythm strip for indications of hyperkalemia (Figure 6-1).
2. Accurate I and O and calculate I/O ratio for fluid balance q 8 and 24 hr.
3. BP, heart rate, and respirations q 4 hr.
4. Temperature q 4 hr.
5. Weigh q AM before breakfast and compare to previous measurements.
6. Assess q 8 hr for positive Trousseau sign by inflating blood pressure cuff for 1 to 5 min inducing carpal spasm and for positive Chvostek sign by tapping the facial nerve just below the temple inducing contraction of the lip, nose, face indicating tetany (hypocalcemia).
7. Auscultate bowel sounds in 4 quadrants for character and frequency of sound q 4 to 8 hr and record onset of high pitched or absent sounds.
8. Assess client for nausea with each contact and record amount and character of emesis.

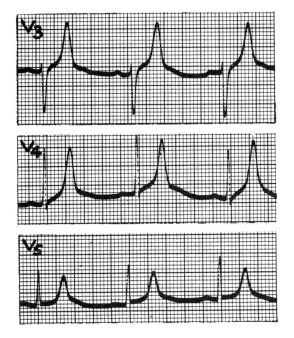

Figure 6-1. Hyperkalemia. Note tall, pointed, "pinched-bottomed" T waves (K = 6.1 mEq/L). Source: Marriot, H.J.L., 1977, with permission.

9. Record amount of each diarrheal stool and describe color and consistency.
10. Auscultate breath sounds in all lung fields q 8 hr and record onset of adventitious sounds.
11. Assess skin color, temperature, moisture, and turgor q 8 hr.
12. Assess client's tolerance for activity and subjective indications of weakness, fatigue, and paresthesia q 4 to 8 hr.
13. Assess LOC q 8 hr and record changes in awareness, orientation, and behavior.
14. Auscultate heart sounds in 4 valvular sites q 8 hr and record onset of extra heart sounds.
15. Palpate peripheral pulses for bilateral quality q 8 hr.
16. Assess for dependent edema q 8 hr.

Monitoring–Interdependent

1. Assess results of laboratory data when available and compare to previous and normal values.
   Serum Potassium: 3.5 to 5.0 mEq/L
   Serum Sodium: 135 to 145 mEq/L

Serum Chloride: 100 to 106 mEq/L
Serum Calcium: 8.5 to 10.5 mg/dl
Serum Phosphate: 3.0 to 4.5 mg/dl
Serum Uric Acid: 3.0 to 7.0 mg/dl
Serum Lactate: 6 to 16 mg/dl
ABGs   pH: 7.35 to 7.45
Po_2: 75 to 100 torr
Pco_2: 35 to 45 torr
HCO_3: 24 to 30 mEq/L
CO_2 Content: 24 to 30 mEq/L
O_2 Saturation: 95 to 100%
BUN: 8 to 25 mg/dl
Creatinine: 0.6 to 1.5 mg/dl
Hematocrit: 45 to 52% males
37 to 48% females
Hemoglobin: 13.0 to 18.0 g/dl males
12.0 to 16.0 g/dl females
Creatinine Clearance: 20 to 26 mg/kg/24 hr male
14 to 22 mg/kg/24 hr female

2. Assess IV site for redness, pain, and swelling q 4 to 8 hr.

Change–Independent

1. Maintain bedrest and minimize activity with serum potassium levels greater than 5.5 mEq/L

2. Maintain adequate hydration with po fluids, if appropriate, depending on fluid status or as prescribed, omitting foods and fluids high in sodium and potassium. (If client in renal failure, po intake will be determined by physician.)

3. Perirectal skin care after each diarrheal stool using protective skin agent to prevent irritation.

4. Apply ice collar to neck with onset of nausea.

5. Mouth care q 4 hr and after each vomiting episode and before meals using appropriate oral antiseptic that is refreshing without tasting too sweet. Once a day, clean teeth with a mixture of H_2O_2 and baking soda to neutralize oral acid and remove plaque.

6. Passive ROME to all major joints while on bedrest q 4 hr.

7. Turn, cough, deep breathe q 2 hr while on bedrest.

8. Back care q 4 hr while on bedrest and massage all bony prominences with lotion.

9. Institute gradual increase in activity when client can tolerate it or when prescribed by physician.

10. O_2 at 2 L/min by nasal cannula if SOB occurs.

11. Assist client to perform ADLs and maintain judicious independence and control over self and environment within physical limitations.
12. Explain condition and progress to client and family with each contact. Assist them to ask questions and express concerns of the present and the future.
13. Include family members in plan of care and allow them to participate, if mutually beneficial.

Change–Interdependent

1. D5W at KVO or as prescribed by physician.
2. Medicate appropriately as prescribed for nausea, diarrhea, and arrhythmias and assess effect in 1 to 30 min.
3. Notify physician if:
    Serum potassium greater than 5.5 mEq/L or less than 3.5 mEq/L during and after therapy
    Serum sodium greater than 145 mEq/L
    Serum calcium less than 8.5 mg/dl
    Serum uric acid greater than 7.0 mg/dl
    Serum lactate greater than 16 mg/dl
    pH is less than 7.3
    BUN greater than 25 mg/dl *and*
    Creatinine greater than 1.5 mg/dl
    EKG changes indicating arrhythmia or presence of tall, peaked T waves
    High pitched or absent bowel sounds with abdominal distention
    Urinary output less than 30 ml/hr or 1500 cc less than intake/24 hr
4. Anticipate physician to prescribe:
    With severe hyperkalemia (usually greater than 7 mEq/L):
        IV calcium chloride 14 mEq (1 amp) or 10% calcium gluconate to antagonize effect of excessive potassium on cell membrane
        IV sodium bicarbonate 44 mEq (1 amp) to correct acidosis
        IV hypertonic glucose (10 to 50%) with insulin to promote intracellular potassium shift
    Kayexalate 15 to 25 g in 50 ml water with 70% sorbitol po or 50 g/200 ml water as enema
    Dialysis if renal failure present or hyperkalemia resistant to other measures
    Lasix to reduce fluid volume overload
    Antiemetics, antidiarrheal medications
    Allopurinol to prevent urinary calculi from high uric acid levels
    Change in chemotherapy dose, rate, or agent

BIBLIOGRAPHY

Corbett, J.V. *Laboratory Tests in Nursing Practice.* Norwalk, Connecticut: Appleton-Century-Crofts, 1982.

Fletcher, B. *Quick Reference to Critical Care Nursing.* Philadelphia: J.B. Lippincott, 1983.

Gordon, M. *Manual of nursing diagnosis.* New York: McGraw-Hill 1982.

Horton, J., and Hill, G.J. *Clinical oncology.* Philadelphia: W.B. Saunders, 1977.

Issacs, M. Life threatening fluid and electrolyte abnormalities in patients with cancer. In A.D. Turnbull (ed.), *Current Problems In Cancer* (vol. 4, no. 3.). Chicago: Year Book Medical Publishers, 1979, pp. 10–11.

Kliger, A.S., and Lovett, D.H. Electrolyte abnormalities in cancer patients. In J. Yarbro and R. Bornstein (eds.), *Oncologic Emergencies.* New York: Grune and Stratton, 1981.

Luckman, J., and Sorensen, K.C. *Medical–Surgical Nursing—A Psychophysiologic Approach* (2nd ed.). Philadelphia: W. B. Saunders, 1980.

Marriott, H.J.L. *Practical Electrocardiography* (6th ed.). Baltimore: Williams & Wilkins, 1977.

Menzel, L.K. Clinical problems of electrolyte balance. *Nursing Clinics of North America,* **15** (3), 1980, 559–576.

Otrakji, J. Disorders of potassium metabolism. *Topics In Emergency Medicine,* **5,** (2), 1983, 53–57.

Otrakji, J. Potassium metabolism disorders. *Critical Care Quarterly,* Aspen Systems Corporation Publishers, 1980, 55–64.

Stolinsky, D.C. Emergencies in oncology—Current management. *The Western Jounral of Medicine,* **129,** (3), 1978, 169–176.

7. Lactic Acidosis

DEFINITION AND CAUSATIVE FACTORS

Lactic acidosis (metabolic acidosis) occurs in the client with cancer when the pH of blood is measured at less than 7.3 and the serum lactic acid concentration is greater than 16 mg/dl. Lactic acidosis results because of rapidly growing malignant cells requiring an increased utilization of glucose producing high concentrations of lactic acid, which may exceed the ability of the liver to metabolize and the kidney to excrete. This is primary lactic acidosis, and it is particularly difficult to correct and often resistant to treatment if the client has liver metastasis, shock, renal failure, or malnutrition. Secondary lactic acidosis is caused by an insufficient delivery of oxygen resulting in hypoxia from tumors restricting the function of the pulmonary system. Normally, the glycolytic pathway has an anaerobic (no oxygen required) phase:

$$Glucose + 8 \text{ reactions} \rightarrow pyruvate$$

and an aerobic (oxygen required) phase:

$$pyruvate \rightarrow acetyl\ CoA \rightarrow Kreb's\ cycle \rightarrow$$

$$oxidative\ phosphorylation \rightarrow ATP + CO_2 + H_2O$$

If hypoxia exists, the pathway ends at pyruvate and lactic acid is the end product, producing lactic acidosis. Primary lactic acidosis is determined by an increased anion gap (normal = 8 to 12 mEq/L), increased serum lactic acid levels (normal = 6 to 8 mg/dl), and a normal oxygen gap (up to 10 torr). If the lactic acidosis is secondary, the oxygen gap would be increased. Hypokalemia would also exist (Chapter 4).

Corresponding cancers include oat cell carcinoma with liver metastasis, acute leukemia, lymphosarcoma, Hodgkin disease, and Burkitt lymphoma. Additional causes of metabolic acidosis include renal failure, severe diarrhea, septicemia, starvation, intestinal malabsorption, ketoacidosis, ingestion of excessive acid substances, anemia, and shock.

ASSESSMENT DATA

- Blood pH less than 7.3 (critical level less than 7.0)
- Decreased plasma bicarbonate level (less than 5 mEq/L is incompatible with life)
- Decreased P_{O_2} level (secondary lactic acidosis only)
- Decreased or normal P_{CO_2}
- Hyperkalemia
- Hyperpnea (compensatory)
- Malaise
- Weakness
- CNS depression with apathy, disorientation, delirium, stupor, coma
- Increased BUN and creatinine indicating renal insufficiency
- Enlarged, nodular liver with liver metastasis or cirrhosis
- Malnutrition
- EKG changes related to hyperkalemia
    tall, thin T waves
    prolonged PR interval
    depressed ST segment
- Cardiac arrhythmias related to hyperkalemia
    bradycardia
    ventricular fibrillation and arrest

NURSING DIAGNOSES

Impaired thought processes, related to changes in LOC, resulting from elevated hydrogen ion concentration in the blood.

Associated Nursing Diagnoses

1. Ineffective breathing pattern, related to inadequate oxygen delivery to the tissues resulting in lactic acidosis.

RATIONALE

Buildup hydrogen ions during anaerobic glycolysis prevents further formation of ATP for energy usage.

Cellular oxidation of glucose is impaired with insufficient oxygen supply.

2. Altered cardiac output, decreased, related to possible life-threatening cardiac arrhythmias, resulting from hyperkalemia.

Depolarization of the membranes of cardiac muscle causes weakness in heart muscle contraction and eventual arrhythmias.

3. Alteration in nutrition, deficit, related to long-term anorexia, nausea, vomiting, contributing to lactic acidosis.

Lack of available glucose necessary for energy formation. Liver dysfunction contributes to insufficient glucose storage.

NURSING INTERVENTIONS

Monitoring–Independent

1. Assess LOC q 2 to 4 hr and record changes in awareness, orientation, and behavior. Record onset of delirium, stupor, or coma.
2. Assess respiratory rate q 2 hr and record depth of inspiration, use of accessory muscles.
3. Assess cardiac rhythm strip for changes indicating hyperkalemia and cardiac arrhythmias q 2 hr and prn.
4. Hourly I and O and calculate I/O ratio for fluid balance q 8 and 24 hr.
5. BP, heart rate, and respirations q 2 hr.
6. Temperature q 4 hr.
7. Assess skin color, temperature, moisture q 4 to 8 hr.
8. Assess client for nausea with each contact and record amount and character of emesis.
9. Assess client's activity tolerance and subjective indications of weakness and fatigue.
10. Auscultate breath sounds in all lung fields q 8 hr and record onset of adventitious sounds.
11. Auscultate heart sounds in 4 valvular sites q 8 hr and record onset of extra heart sounds.
12. Auscultate bowel sounds in 4 quadrants q 8 hr and record pitch and frequency of sound.
13. Palpate peripheral pulses for bilateral quality q 8 hr.
14. Inspect all dependent areas for edema q 8 hr.
15. Weight q AM before breakfast and record (information necessary for bicarbonate therapy).

Monitoring–Interdependent

1. Assess laboratory data; when available; and compare to previous and normal values.

   ABGs   pH: 7.35 to 7.45
   P_{O_2}: 75 to 100 torr
   P_{CO_2}: 35 to 45 torr
   HCO_3: 24 to 30 mEq/L
   CO_2 Content: 24 to 30 mEq/L
   O_2 Saturation: 95 to 100%
   Serum Sodium: 135 to 145 mEq/L
   Serum Potassium: 3.5 to 5.0 mEq/L
   Serum Chloride: 100 to 106 mEq/L
   Serum Lactate: 6 to 16 mg/dl
   Bun: 8 to 25 mg/dl
   Creatinine: 0.6 to 1.5 mg/dl
   Hemoglobin: 13.0 to 18.0 g/dl males
                 12.0 to 16.0 g/dl females
   Hematocrit: 45 to 52% males
                 37 to 48% females
   Liver Function Tests
   Creatinine Clearance: 20 to 26 mg/kg/24 hr males
                          14 to 22 mg/kg/24 hr females
   Urine pH: 4.6 to 8.0 (average = 6.0)

2. Assess IV site for redness, pain, swelling q 4 to 8 hr.

3. Assess client for overcorrection of acidosis by:
   Blood pH greater than 7.45
   Shallow, slow respirations—compensatory
   Hypokalemia
   Irritability, belligerence followed by lethargy and coma
   Urine pH greater than 7.0

Change–Independent

1. Maintain bedrest with HOB at level of maximum comfort and minimize activity with blood pH less than 7.3

2. O_2 at 2 L/min by nasal cannula if P_{O_2} less than 70 torr or as prescribed by physician.

3. Reorient to time, place, and reason for hospitalization q 1 to 2 hr when changes in LOC occur.

4. Offer fluids to 120 ml q 1 hr while awake, alternating between fat free milk and lemonade or grape juice (less acid, low potassium), if client can tolerate po fluids and is not in renal failure, or NPO.

5. Mouth care q 4 hr using soft toothbrush and an oral antiseptic. Once a day, clean teeth with a mixture of H_2O_2 and baking soda to neutralize oral acid and remove plaque.

6. Perirectal skin care after each diarrheal stool using protective skin agent to prevent irritation.

7. Passive ROME to all major joints while on bedrest q 4 hr.

8. Turn, cough, deep breathe q 2 hr while on bedrest.

9. Back care q 4 hr while on bedrest and massage all bony prominences with lotion.

10. Reorient to time, place, reason for hospitalization with each contact if client confused or disoriented.

11. Institute gradual increase in activity when client can tolerate it or when prescribed by physician.

12. Assist client to perform ADLs and maintain judicious independence and control over self and environment within physical limitations.

13. Explain condition and progress to client and family with each contact. Assist them to ask questions and express concerns of the present and the future.

14. Include family members in plan of care and allow them to participate, if mutually beneficial.

Change—Interdependent

1. D5W at KVO or as prescribed by physician.

2. Medicate appropriately for nausea, vomiting, diarrhea, and cardiac arrhythmias as prescribed and assess effect in 1 to 30 min.

3. Notify physician if:
   Blood pH less than 7.3 or greater than 7.5 during or after treatment
   Po_2 less than 70 torr
   Pco_2 less than 35 torr
   HCO_3 less than 24 mEq/L
   CO_2 content less than 24 mEq/L
   Serum potassium greater than 5.5 mEq/L or less than 3.0 mEq/L during or after treatment
   Serum calcium less than 8.5 mg/dl
   Serum lactate acid greater than 16 mg/dl
   BUN greater than 25 mg/dl *and*
   Creatinine greater than 1.6 mg/dl
   Hemoglobin less than 30 g/dl
   EKG changes indicating hyperkalemia
   Life-threatening cardiac arrhythmias
   Urinary output less than 30 ml/hr or 1000 cc less than intake/24 hr

4. Consult with physician concerning need for hyperalimentation or TPN if client has experienced long-term anorexia, vomiting, or diarrhea. (Protein or fat catabolism exacerbates lactic acidosis, and if the client is in renal failure, special mixtures can be used to maintain protein restriction required in renal failure [Chapter 39]).

5. Anticipate physician to prescribe:

IV $NaHCO_3$ to correct acidosis according to:

$$mEq \ NaHCO_3 = 0.5 \times kg \ body \ wt \times (desired \ HCO_3 \ minus \ measured \ HCO_3)$$

or

$$mEq \ NaHCO_3 = \frac{Base \ deficit \ (mEq/L) \times kg \ body \ wt}{4}$$

Correction of hyperkalemia*

1 amp 10% calcium chloride IV, hypertonic glucose (10 to 50%) with insulin, Kayexalate in sorbitol by mouth or in water as enema

Dialysis if renal failure present

Bicarbonate po with mild chronic lactic acidosis

Dichloroacetate to oxidize lactate to acetyl CoA and CO_2 if hypoxia corrected or absent

---

BIBLIOGRAPHY

Corbett, J.V. *Laboratory Tests in Nursing Practice*. Norwalk, Connecticut: Appleton-Century-Crofts, 1982.

De Vita, V.T., Hellman, S., and Rosenberg, S.A. *Cancer, Principles and Practice of Oncology*. Philadelphia: J.B. Lippincott, 1982.

Done, A.K. The toxic emergency. *Emergency Medicine,* 13(10), 1981, 68–84.

Fields, A.L.A., Wolman, S.L., and Halperin, M.L. Chronic lactic acidosis in a patient with cancer: Therapy and metabolic consequences. *Cancer,* 47(8), 1981, 2026–2029.

Gordon, M. *Manual of Nursing Diagnosis*. New York: McGraw-Hill, 1982.

---

*Careful monitoring of serum potassium levels is required. If the acidosis is corrected, potassium will shift into the cells and hypokalemia may result. With adequate kidney function, potassium is being excreted in an attempt to compensate, which further compounds the problem. The physician may prescribe IV potassium to be added to IV fluids anticipating this to occur.

Guthrie, H.A. *Introductory Nutrition* (4th ed.). St. Louis: C.V. Mosby, 1979.

Hobbs, J. Metabolic acidosis. *afp Practical Therapeutics*, **23**(2), 1981, 220-227.

Kliger, A.S., and Lovett, D.H. Electrolyte abnormalities in cancer patients. In J. Yarbro and R. Bornstein (eds.), *Oncologic Emergencies*. New York: Grune and Stratton, 1981.

Luckman, J., and Sorensen, K.C. *Medical-Surgical Nursing—A Psychophysiologic Approach* (2nd ed.). Philadelphia: W.B. Saunders, 1980.

Wallach, J. *Interpretation of Diagnostic Tests* (2nd ed.) Boston: Little, Brown, 1974.

8. Secretion of Inappropriate Antidiuretic Hormone

DEFINITION AND CAUSATIVE FACTORS

Secretion of inappropriate antidiuretic hormone (SIADH) is a syndrome characterized by extracellular hypoosmolality, water intoxication, hyponatremia, natriuria, normovolemia, urine osmolality greater than appropriate for plasma osmolality (hypertonic to plasma) and normal renal and adrenal function. This syndrome occurs in the client with cancer because of the constant release of ADH from the posterior pituitary which becomes impervious to the usual feedback control mechanisms. Normally, ADH is released from the posterior pituitary gland when the plasma osmolality increases or the plasma volume decreases causing greater water reabsorption in the collecting ducts of the nephron producing a concentrated and decreased urine volume. Pain, stress, trauma, hemorrhage, certain drugs (morphine, barbituates, thiazides, vincristine, and cyclophosphamide), as well as certain malignancies also stimulate the release of ADH. The osmolality of plasma is held constant within a range of 286 to 294 mOsm/kg of water and the osmolality of urine usually reflects that of the plasma. When the plasma osmolality decreases or the plasma volume increases, ADH is inhibited and the urine volume becomes greater and more dilute.

The client with SIADH usually does not become symptomatic until the serum sodium level is 120 mEq/L or less, and the neurologic symptoms will occur at 110 mEq/L. Hyponatremia has two stages: initially, there is an early dilutional hyponatremia because of water retention, followed by an excessive sodium excretion most probably related to increased circulating volume and glomular filtration rate and decreased aldosterone secretion. SIADH occurs in the client with cancer because the malignant cells of certain cancers—bronchogenic, oat cell, pancreas, and Hodgkin—have the ability to synthesize, store, and release ADH.

Corresponding cancers include lung, pancreas, duodenum, brain, esophagus, colon, ovary, larnyx, acute and chronic leukemia, mesothelioma, reticulum-cell sarcoma, prostate, bronchus, nasopharynx, Hodgkin, thymoma, and lymphosarcoma. Tuberculosis, bacterial pneumonia, lung abscess, CHF, renal failure, liver disease with ascites, diabetic acidosis, meningitis, brain abscess, head injury, Addison disease, and hypothyroidism are additional causes. Drug related SIADH include vincristine, cyclophosphamide, thiazide diuretics, carbamazepine, oxytocin, acetaminophen, and chlofibrate.

ASSESSMENT DATA

- Hyponatremia—serum sodium less than 130 mEq/L
- Serum osmolality less than 280 mOsm/kg
- Normovolemia
- Increased sodium excretion greater than 20 mEq/L
- Increased urine osmolality greater that 500 mOsm/kg
- Normal renal and adrenal function
- Absence of edema

- With serum sodium levels less than 110 mEq/L
  Personality changes
  Weight gain
  Weakness
  Anorexia, nausea, vomiting
  Lethargy
  Seizures
  Coma
- Decreased BUN and creatinine
- Hypokalemia and hypocalcemia—probably dilutional

NURSING DIAGNOSES

Alteration in fluid volume, excess, related to serum hyponatremia and hypoosmolality of plasma producing water intoxication.

RATIONALE

Certain cancers maintain the ability to synthesize, store, and release ADH, thus causing excessive retention of water.

NURSING INTERVENTIONS

Monitoring–Independent

1. Accurate I and O and calculate I/O ratio for fluid balance q 8 and 24 hr.
2. Assess LOC q 4 hr and record changes in awareness, orientation, and behavior.
3. Auscultate breath sounds in all lung fields q 8 hr and record onset of adventitious sounds.
4. Assess skin color, temperature, and moisture q 8 hr.
5. Weigh q AM before breakfast and compare to previous weight.
6. Oral temperature q 4 hr.

7. Urine specific gravity q 4 to 8 hr.
8. Assess client for subjective and objective indications of fatigue and weakness q 8 hr.
9. BP, heart rate, and respirations q 4 hr.
10. Auscultate heart sounds in 4 valvular sites q 8 hr and record onset of gallop.
11. Palpate peripheral pulses for bilateral quality q 8 hr.
12. Assess dependent areas for edema q 8 hr.
13. Assess client for nausea or vomiting with each contact and for anorexia at meal times.

Note: Although SIADH does NOT cause edema, there are other types of conditions involving hyponatremia that do, and until SIADH has been definitely established, all parameters involving hyponatremia and fluid volume should be assessed.

Monitoring–Interdependent

1. Assess laboratory data when available and compare to previous and normal values.
   Serum Osmolality: 286 to 294 mOsm/kg
   Urine Osmolality: 50 to 1200 mOsm/kg (200 to 800 average)
   Serum Sodium: 135 to 145 mEq/L
   Serum Chloride: 100 to 106 mEq/L
   Serum Potassium: 3.5 to 4.5 mEq/L
   Serum Calcium: 8.5 to 10.5 mg/dl
   BUN: 8 to 25 mg/dl
   Creatinine: 0.6 to 1.5 mg/dl
   Urine Sodium: 40 to 220 mEq/L/24 hr
2. Assess results of water-load test (Boh, D.M. and VanSon, A., 1982).
   Obtain current weight, serum sodium, potassium, chloride, creatinine, BUN, and osmolality of serum and urine and record.
   Note: This test should not be done unless client's serum sodium level is 125 mEq/L or more. Used to assist in diagnosis of SIADH.
   Instruct client to:
   Remain flat in bed
   Maintain NPO 12 hrs before and throughout test (5 to 6 hr)
   Abstain from smoking (nicotine increases ADH secretion) 12 hrs before and throughout test
   Use urinal or bedpan throughout test
   Administer 300 ml of water 1 hr prior to test to replace insensible loss
   Administer 20 ml water/kg body weight
   Collect urine for 5 hr

Calculate urine volume and specific gravity
Send urine specimen to laboratory for osmolality
3. Assess client for nausea, abdominal fullness, fatigue, SOB, and chest pain throughout test period
   Normal results
      80% of water excreted in 5 hr
      Urine Osmolality: 100 to 1000 mOsm/kg
      Specific Gravity: 1.015 to 1.025

Change–Independent

1. Maintain bedrest with minimized activity with serum sodium level less than 120 mEq/L.
2. Turn, cough, deep breathe q 2 hr while on bedrest.
3. Bathe, without soap, using commercially prepared bath emollient bid.
4. Apply ice collar to neck with onset of nausea.
5. Back care and massage all bony prominences with lotion q 4 hr.
6. Mouth care using soft toothbrush and oral antiseptic q 4 hr or after meals. Once a day clean teeth with a mixture of H_2O_2 and baking soda to neutralize oral acid and remove plaque.
7. Passive ROME to all major joints q 4 hr while on bedrest.
8. Institute all safety measures. Keep side rails up and pad if client restless or disoriented, place call light and personal articles within easy reach, and ambulate with assistance.
9. Reorient to time, place, reason for hospitalization with each contact if client confused or disoriented.
10. Before all procedures, explain purpose and technique in understandable terms.
11. Assist client to perform ADLs and maintain judicious independence over self and environment within physical limitations.
12. Explain condition and progress to client and family with each contact. Assist to ask questions and express concerns of the present and the future.
13. Include family members in plan of care and allow them to participate, if mutually beneficial.

Change–Interdependent

1. Notify physician if:
      Serum sodium less than 120 mEq/L
      Serum potassium less than 3.5 mEq/L
      Serum calcium less than 8.5 mEq/L
      Serum osmolality less than 280 mOsm/kg

Changes occur in LOC
Weight gain greater than 1 to 2 kg/day

2. Anticipate physician to prescribe:

Water restriction (intake = output) in mild cases

3% Normal saline IV to restore serum sodium

Lasix 1 mg/kg body weight to produce hypotonic diuresis. Hypertonic saline increases serum sodium levels and fluid volume but also stimulates the kidney to excrete sodium. Lasix prevents this by eliminating excess water.

Demeclocycline or lithium carbonate in chronic SIADH to interfere with the action of ADH on the collecting tubule of the nephron. Assess client for signs and symptoms of nephrotoxicity and sunlight sensitivity with the administration of demeclocycline.

Discontinue or reduce vincristine and cyclophosphamide chemotherapy.

Drug dosages must be reduced in clients with SIADH:

- Penicillin
- Cephalosporins
- Tetracycline
- NegGram
- Furadantin
- Digoxin
- Pronestyl
- Thiazide diuretics
- Morphine Sulfate

- Barbiturates
- Nipride
- Dilantin
- Aspirin
- Phenobarbital
- Isuprel Hydrochloride
- Orinase
- Diabinese

BIBLIOGRAPHY

Boh, D.M. and VanSon, A. The Water-Load Test. *AJN*, **82**(1), 1982, 112–113.

Clinch, D. Syndrome of inappropriate antidiuretic hormone secretion associated with stress. *Lancet*, **1**(8275), 1982, 1131–1132.

Corbett, J.V. *Laboratory Tests in Nursing Practice*. Norwalk, Connecticut: Appleton-Century-Crofts, 1982.

Decaux, G., Unger, J., Brimiouile, S., and Mockel, J. Hyponatremia in the syndrome of inappropriate secretion of antidiuretic hormone. *The Journal of the American Medical Association*, **247**(4), 1982, 471–474.

Franco, L.M. Syndrome of inappropriate secretion of antidiuretic hormone. *Journal of Neurosurgical Nursing*, **14**(5), 1982, 276–279.

Gordon, M. *Manual of Nursing Diagnosis*. New York: McGraw-Hill, 1982.

Hamburger, S., and Rush, D. Syndrome of inappropriate secretion of antidiuretic hormone. *Critical Care Quarterly*, Aspen Systems Corporation, 1980, pp. 119–129.

Horton, J., and Hill, G.J. *Clinical Oncology*. Philadelphia: W.B. Saunders, 1977.

Kliger, A.S., and Lovett, D.H. Electrolyte abnormalities in cancer patients. In J. Yarbro and R. Bornstein (eds.), *Oncologic Emergencies*. New York: Grune and Stratton, 1981, pp. 215–220.

Yasko, J.M. Syndrome of inappropriate antidiuretic hormone secretion. In J.M. Yasko (ed.), *Guidelines for Cancer Care: Symptom Management*. Virginia: Reston, 1983, 362–366.

9. Postmastectomy Lymphedema

Lymphedema occurs in the postmastectomy client as a result of axillary node dissection, a lack of collateral lymphatic circulation, and nonaggressive or inconsistent intervention. The incidence of lymphedema varies among authors, but 30 to 60% appears to be the concensus—10% of these are severe. Lymphedema can be transient, occurring within 6 weeks after surgery and self-limiting, or latent, occurring months or years after surgery and chronic (Fig. 9-1). Normally, lymph flow depends on the lymphatic pump involving valvular and muscle compression mechanisms of propulsion and an equilibrium between interstitial and lymphatic capillary fluid pressure. Lymph absorption depends on lymph formation, equilibrium between lymphatic capillary pressure and filtration, and lymphatic capillary permeability. Lymphedema develops because of lymphatic capillary obstruction, lymphatic statis, and changes in lymphatic circulatory pressures.

Lymphatic obstruction → increased hydrostatic pressure → lymph vessel dilatation → valvular incompetency → statis → increased protein concentration → proliferation of fibroblasts → bacterial growth → infection → inflammation and thrombosis plus increased lymphatic permeability → edema

The primary causes of lymphatic obstruction are surgical interruption, neoplastic invasion or emboli, radiation, thrombophlebitis (lymph contains clotting factors), and immobility. Lymphedema can result in loss of arm function, cellulitis, lymphangitis, and compartment syndrome.

Corresponding cancers include breast and neoplastic invasion of lymph vessels, capillaries, or nodes. Hypoproteinemia, radiation scarring, obesity, immobility, and infection are additional causes.

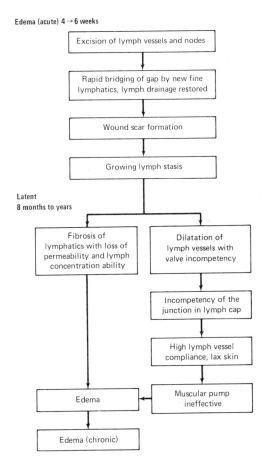

Edema (acute) 4 → 6 weeks

Latent
8 months to years

Figure 9-1. Mechanisms of transient and latent lymphedema.

ASSESSMENT DATA

- Edema of arm measuring greater than 4 cm as compared to unaffected arm
- Lymphadenopathy
- Shiny and translucent skin
- Skin cold to touch
- Tenderness

- Decrease or absence of pulses
- Significant weight gain
- Jugular vein distention
- Limited ROM and pain with ROM
- Paresthesia
- Albumin level less than 3.7 g/dl

NURSING DIAGNOSES	RATIONALE

Alteration in tissue perfusion, related to lymphatic fluid accumulation in surrounding tissues, resulting in an interference of cellular O_2–CO_2 exchange and cellular death.

Increased concentration of protein and/or bacterial agents in the lymphatic vessels and a decrease in the net flow of capillary permeability.

Associated Nursing Diagnoses

1. Impaired physical mobility, related to an edematous extremity that has lost its ability for muscular function and activity.

   Decreased propulsion of lymph through vessels causes stasis resulting in accumulation of lymphatic fluid.

2. Potential for physical injury, related to the loss of tactile, sensory, and motor function, as a result of edema.

   Chronic venous stasis yields edema. Stimulation of sympathetic nerve fibers of the skin causes vasodilatation and localized edema.

3. Disturbances in self-concept, related to a change in body image, resulting from an enlarged, misshapened, edematous arm and a loss of a breast.

   Physical body alterations demand reaction of an individual to his or her self and environment.

NURSING INTERVENTIONS

Monitoring–Independent

1. Measure edematous extremity qd in cm and compare to nonedematous extremity using predetermined landmarks of the wrist and 6 cm below and above elbow, and record.
2. Palpate both axilla qd and record number, location, consistency, moveability of each node, and the size of the largest nodule.
3. Inspect affected arm for color, temperature, discoloration, translucency, skin breakdown, and areas of necrosis q 8 hr.
4. Determine nail blanching time of affected arm q 6 hr and record in seconds.
5. Assess affected arm for tenderness on palpation and pain with ROM movement q 8 hr.

6. Assess for pulse deficit in affected arm q 8 hr. (Auscultate apical heart rate and palpate radial pulse counting number of missed beats.)
7. Palpate radial and brachial pulses in affected arm for rate and intensity q 8 hr and compare to unaffected arm.
8. Assess sensory function of affected arm q 8 hr using sharp or dull side of pin and object identification.
9. Assess muscle grip and movement on command of all parts of arm, hand, and fingers in affected arm q 8 hr and compare to unaffected arm.
10. Assess for disturbances in kinesis by Romberg test (swaying that occurs when client stands with feet together and arms at side) q 8 hr.
11. Weigh qd before breakfast and compare to previous measurement.
12. Accurate I and O and calculate I/O ratio for fluid balance q 8 and 24 hr.
13. Assess neck vein distention and record in cm q 8 hr with HOB at 45 to 60°.
14. Oral temperature q 4 hr.
15. BP, heart rate, respirations q 4 hr.
16. Auscultate breath sounds in all lung fields, symmetry of chest expansion, and use of accessory muscles q 8 hr and record onset of adventitious sounds (lymphedema can result in fluid overload).

Monitoring–Interdependent

1. Assess laboratory data when available and compare to previous and normal values.
   Serum Albumin: 3.5 to 5.0 g/dl
   WBC: 4,500 to 11,500/mm^3
   Serum Sodium: 135 to 145 mEq/L
   Serum Potassium: 3.5 to 5.0 mEq/L
   Serum Chloride: 100 to 106 mEq/L
   Serum Calcium: 8.5 to 10.5 mg/dl

Change–Independent

1. Elevate affected arm on a pillow above apex of heart at all times.
2. Massage affected arm while elevated starting at the wrist and advancing to the shoulder q 4 hr (compression and stroking increases lymph flow).
3. Institute progressive exercise plan immediately postoperative mastectomy.
   AROME to all unaffected extremities q 4 hr.
   AROME to all joints of affected arm qid to point of pain, resistance, or fatigue.

Gradual raising of affected arm bid.

Hand-alternating clinch with extending and flexing fingers q 2 hr for 10 min gradually increasing to 20 to 30 min.

Rope pulley exercises beginning with 2 to 3 times q 8 hr.

Wall climbing finger exercises beginning with 2 to 3 times q alternate 8 hr.

Increase each exercise by 1 to 2 times more each day depending on pain threshold.

4. Teach exercise plan to client and family and devise Check Flow Sheet of type of exercise, date, time, and duration to illustrate progress (Table 9-1).

5. Apply arm sling to assist in body equilibrium for sitting, standing, or walking.

6. Eliminate trauma to affected arm by:

Using sheep skin, air mattress, side rail padding

Posting signs "No venipunctures, BP, or tourniquets in (right or left) arm" on client's door and HOB

Removing all chemical irritants—alcohol, etc.

Preventing heat or cold applications or contact including matches, cigarettes

Filing fingernails to shortest possible length

Removing all heavy jewelry capable of scratching, bruising, or constricting affected extremity

Preventing overuse of affected arm. After exercising, inspect arm for pallor or other adverse signs and change exercise frequency and duration

7. Massage affected arm and all bony prominences with lotion q 8 hr after washing in tepid water and pat drying.

8. Assist client to express feelings of anger, hostility, shame, anxiety, depression, change in body image, and loss of femininity by being astute to verbal and nonverbal cues and using therapeutic communication skills. *Do not be tempted to convey the message that it is better to have a breast removed than to die of cancer!*

9. Assist client to perform ADLs and maintain independence and control over self and environment within physical limitations.

10. Explain condition and progress to client and family with each contact. Assist them to ask questions and express concerns of the present and the future.

11. Include family members in plan of care and allow them to participate, if mutually beneficial.

Change–Interdependent

1. Measure affected arm for stocking hose (TED, Jobst) if prescribed. It should be just tight enough to create a pressure to increase tissue perfusion and venous blood flow by compressing the walls of the veins. This prevents dilatation of the veins, venous stasis, and edema. The stocking comes in three varieties. One type is applied from the dorsum of the hand, wraps between the thumb and forefinger, and extends up to the deltoid muscle; the second extends from midwrist to deltoid muscle; and the third extends from the dorsum of the hand and has a shoulder attachment that straps around the back and attaches in the front. The type used will be determined by the physician. All are worn from morning until bedtime, and are applied before getting out of bed so that gravity does not have a chance to increase the swelling. Some clients may need to wear it less frequently depending on the amount and cause of their lymphedema. As with any hose, assess extremities for cyanosis and blanching as signs of being too tight. Also, assess for being too loose as a new size may be needed.
2. Applied mechanical pressure pump if prescribed q 2 to 3 hr.
3. Discuss with physician referral to Reach for Recovery and obtaining a volunteer.
4. Medicate 30 min to 1 hr prior to exercises as prescribed and assess effect in 10 to 20 min.

PRECAUTIONS

The following hints are given to help clients with arm care after mastectomy and to prevent injury and infection.

To prevent burns:
   Use padded mitts when using the oven, grill, or fireplace.
   Tan slowly to prevent sunburn. Utilize sunscreens that contain PABA.

To prevent trapping of more fluid in the arm because of pressure:
   Stop smoking. Tobacco use causes vasoconstriction.
   Carry purse, packages, suitcases, and other heavy objects on the unaffected side.
   Wear watch and jewelry on the unaffected arm.
   Avoid clothes with tight sleeves or those with elastic in the sleeves.
   Prevent anyone from taking a blood pressure on the affected side.
   Do not let the arm hang limply at the side.
   Wear elastic sleeve regularly if your surgeon has prescribed one.

TABLE 9-1. EXERCISE FLOW SHEET

Date	Ball Squeeze q 2 hr	Rope Pulley 10A/6P/10A	Finger Climb 8A/4P/8P	Arm Raise 12P/2P	Other/ Comments	Arm Circumference (in.)
7/25	5 min	2 times	1 time	$\frac{1}{2}$ up	Pain severe	8
7/26	5 min	3 times	2 times	$\frac{1}{2}$ up	Pain mod.	8 $\frac{1}{2}$
7/27						
7/28						
7/29						
7/30						
7/31						
8/1						
8/2	30	10	8	All	Mild	8 $\frac{1}{4}$

To prevent cuts, scratches, and irritation:

Wear heavy gloves while gardening, and avoid thorny plants.

Wear a thimble while sewing.

Use an electric shaver to shave underarm of affected extremity.

Keep hands and cuticles soft with regular use (three times daily) of hand cream. Gently push cuticle back when applying hand cream; never cut cuticle. If hands become very dry during cold weather, apply hand cream and wear cotton gloves while sleeping.

Always wear gloves outside in cold weather.

Prevent all injections (flu shots, vaccinations, medications) from being given in the affected arm.

Prohibit the taking of blood from the affected arm.

Wear lined rubber gloves when washing dishes or doing household cleaning.

Wear protective equipment when participating in appropriate sports.

Open mail with letter opener.

Use a mild deodorant on the affected side.

Immediately wash even the slightest cut, cleanse thoroughly, and apply a Band-Aid.

Call a physician if arm becomes hot, red, or swollen.

Carry a card or wear a Medic-Alert tag that indicates Lymphedema Arm—No Tests—No Hypos.

BIBLIOGRAPHY

Bates, B. *A guide to physical examination.* Philadelphia: J.B. Lippincott, 1974.

Burns, N. *Nursing and cancer.* Philadelphia: W.B. Saunders, 1982.

Corbett, J.V. *Laboratory tests in nursing practice.* Norwalk, Connecticut: Appleton-Century-Crofts, 1982.

Gordon, M. *Manual of nursing diagnosis.* New York: McGraw-Hill, 1982.

Lupien, A. Head-off compartment syndrome before it's too late. *RN*, **43**(6), 1980, 39–41.

Markowski, J., Wilcox, J.P., and Helm, P.A. Lymphedema incidence after specific postmastectomy therapy. *Archives of Physical Medical Rehabilitation*, **62**, 1981, 449–451.

Olszewski, W. On the pathomechanism of developing postmastectomy lymphedema. *Lymphology*, **6**, 1973, 35–51.

Yoffey, J.M., and Courtice, F.C. *Lymphatics, lymph and the lymphomyeloid complex.* New York: Academic Press, 1970.

PART II
HEMODYNAMICS

10. Thrombocytopenia

Thrombocytopenia is a decrease in circulating platelets (thrombocytes) necessary for the blood clotting mechanism. Platelets function in clot formation by being trapped in the fibrin network at the site of blood vessel injury.

1. Vascular injury $\longrightarrow$ release of tissue thromboplastin
2. Thromboplastin + 7 factors + prothrombin $\longrightarrow$ thrombin
3. Thrombin + fibrinogin $\longrightarrow$ fibrin
4. Fibrin + platelets $\longrightarrow$ clot formation

Thrombocytopenia is the most common cause of bleeding in the client with cancer. It is a result of metastatic infiltration of bone marrow decreasing the production of the platelet precursor megakaryocytes, depression of bone marrow from chemotherapy and radiation, and the abnormal destruction of platelets by the spleen or antibody production in lymphoma and leukemia.

Thrombocytopenia is defined as less than 100,000 per cu mm. Normal values are 130,000 to 370,000 mm^3. With a decrease to 20,000 to 50,000 cu mm, there is a potential risk of bleeding, but if less than 20,000 mm^3, spontaneous bleeding can occur. These values differ among authors, but the total condition of the client must be considered rather than numbers. Petechia and bruising are characteristic of thrombocytopenia. Petechiae occur with injury to the microcirculation and are most frequently observed initially in the distal arms and legs or under blood pressure cuffs and tourniquets. Bruising is caused by injury to larger blood vessels resulting in leakage into surrounding tissue—a major cause in intracranial hemorrhage.

Corresponding cancers include acute and chronic lymphocytic leukemia, Hodgkin and non-Hodgkin lymphomas. DIC, hypersplenism, liver dysfunction, myelosuppression (L-asparaginase or mithramycin induced), radiation, and high-dose pencillin are additional causes.

ASSESSMENT DATA

- Platelet count less than 50,000 mm^3
- Petechia
- Bruises
- Mucous membrane bleeding—gums, vagina, nose, GI tract
- Hematomas
- Menorrhagia, metrorrhagia
- Hematemesis, melena
- Recent alcohol consumption, thiazide diuretics, ASA, anticoagulant, or Indocin therapy.
- Indication of intracranial bleeding, visual disturbances, loss of motor function, change in LOC, headache, or change in pupil equality
- Decreased hemoglobin and hematocrit levels

NURSING DIAGNOSES

RATIONALE

Potential alteration in cardiac output, decreased, related to a decrease in platelets necessary for clot formation thereby increasing the risk of bleeding and hemorrhage.

Decreased clot formation causes a loss of blood volume in the circulation, resulting in a decreased cardiac output.

Associated Nursing Diagnoses
1. Alterations in tissue perfusion, decreased, related to insufficient blood supply to vital organs, resulting in impairment or loss of function.

Multiple physiological injury will occur after body compensatory mechanisms have been exhausted due to thrombocytopenia.

NURSING INTERVENTIONS

Monitoring–Independent

1. BP, heart rate, respirations q 15 min to 1 hr during acute bleeds, q 2 to 4 hr with platelet count less than 100,000 mm^3.
2. Assess skin for color, temperature, moisture, petechia, or bruising q 4 to 8 hr.
3. Inspect gums, oral cavity, and conjunctiva for bleeding q 4 to 8 hr.

4. Hemocult all emesis, stools, and urine and NG tube drainage (if applicable) q 4 to 8 hrs.
5. Assess LOC, behavior, pupil size and equality, and motor function q 4 to 8 hr.
6. Pad count and describe saturation with menstruation, vaginal bleeds, or rectal bleeds.
7. Auscultate heart sounds in 4 valvular sites q 8 hr and document changes in rate, rhythm, or onset of gallop.
8. Auscultate bowel sounds in 4 quadrants and assess abdomen for rebound tenderness, firmness, and distention q 4 to 8 hr.
9. Auscultate lung sounds in all fields, symmetry of chest expansion, and use of accessory muscles q 4 to 8 hr.
10. Hourly I and O and calculate I/O ratio for fluid balance q 8 and 24 hr.
11. Assess all venipuncture sites, IM sites, or other skin integrity alterations for oozing or subcutaneous bleeding for 30 min.
12. Palpate peripheral pulses for bilateral quality q 8 hr.
13. Assess IV site for redness, swelling, and pain q 4 to 8 hr.

Monitoring–Interdependent

1. Assess laboratory data when available and compare to previous and normal values.

	NORMS	THROMBOCYTOPENIA
Platelet count	130,000–370,000 mm^3	<100,000 mm^3
Fibrinogen	200–500 mg/dl	Decreased
Hemoglobin	13–18.0 g/dl males	Decreased
	12–16.0 g/dl females	Decreased
Hematocrit	45–52% males	Decreased
	37–48% females	Decreased

RBC: 4.6 to 6.2 $\times$ 10^6/mm^3 males
        4.2 to 5.4 $\times$ 10^6/mm^3 females
MCH: 27 to 32 pg
MCHC: 32 to 36%
MCV: 80 to 94 cu microns
WBC: 4,500 to 11,500/mm^3

2. Question use of aspirin, anticoagulants, thiazide diuretics, unnecessary catheters, or excessive laboratory work.
3. With platelet administration:
   Blood pressure q 15 to 30 min during infusion, q 1 to 2 hr $\times$6 after administration

Assess for hives, chills, fever. Do not discontinue but slow infusion rate and notify physican. Use gauze when removing IV devices instead of alcohol (causes local vasodilatation deterring clot formation). Platelets should be infused rapidly and within 1 hr after obtaining from donor. They are not HLA matched so that allergic reactions can occur. Sibling donors are best to prevent reactions.

Change–Independent

1. Apply pressure to all venipuncture sites for 10 min or until bleeding stops.
2. Place sandbags over site of bone marrow aspiration or biopsy.
3. Coordinate all laboratory work so that venipunctures are minimized.
4. Use smallest gauge needles appropriate to IV infusions and parenteral injections.
5. File fingernails as short as possible and use soft brush to clean every day.
6. Force fluids to 120 ml 1 hr while awake, if applicable.
7. Bedrest with minimized activity if platelet count less than 50,000 mm^3.
8. Passive ROM to all major joints q 8 hr if tolerated while on bedrest.
9. Turn, cough, deep breathe q 2 hr.
10. Light massage using nonastringent lotions to all bony prominences q 4 hr.
11. Oral and teeth care using sponge tip applicators and half strength H_2O_2 q 8 hr. Once a day, clean teeth with H_2O_2 and baking soda mixed into a paste to neutralize mouth acid and remove plaque.
12. Bathe, without soap, using commercially prepared bath emollient qd.
13. Eliminate all environmental hazards to safety. Keep side rails up and pad if client restless or disoriented; put bed in low position, and place call light and personal articles within easy reach.
14. Reorient to time, place, reason for hospitalization with each contact if client confused or disoriented.
15. Assist client to perform ADLs and maintain judicious independence and control over self and environment within physical limitations.
16. Explain condition and progress to client and family with each contact. Assist them to ask questions and express concerns of the present and the future.
17. Include family members to participate in plan of care, if mutually therapeutic.
18. Teach client to (if applicable):
    Eliminate nose trauma from blowing, picking
    Eliminate valsalva maneuver by consciously preventing straining during defecation or holding breath when changing position

Seek assistance when ambulating or performing ADLs

Do NOT use dental floss, toothpicks, tampons

19. Before all procedures explain purpose and technique in understandable terms.

Change–Interdependent

1. D5W at KVO or as prescribed by physician.

2. Notify physician if:
   Platelet count less than 50,000 mm^3
   Hemaglobin less than 10 g/dl
   Hematocrit less than 30%
   BP systolic 90 torr or less
   Active and profuse bleeding occurs from any site

3. Anticipate the physician to prescribe:
   Nose packs soaked in adrenalin or thrombin for epistaxis to constrict superficial blood vessels
   Medroxyprogesterone q week and Premarin qd to stop uterine bleeding
   Ice water lavages until clear for gastric bleeding
   Platelet transfusions (4 to 10 units) if platelet count 20,000 or less or if active bleeding occurs with platelet count critically less than 100,000 mm^3
   Stool softener and antacids to decrease GI irritation

4. Consult with dietitian and physician concerning need for high protein, high calorie foods and liquids.

5. No IM injections or suppositories.

BIBLIOGRAPHY

Corbett, J.V. *Laboratory tests in nursing practice.* Norwalk, Connecticut: Appleton-Century-Crofts, 1982.

Gannon, C.T. Bleeding due to thrombocytopenia. In J.M. Yasko (Ed.), *Guidelines for cancer care—Symptom management.* Virginia: Reston, 1983, pp. 25-32.

Gordon, M. *Manual of nursing diagnosis.* New York: McGraw-Hill, 1982.

Harvey, A.M., Johns, R.J., McKusick, V.A., Owens, A.H., Jr., and Ross, R.S. *The principles and practice of medicine* (20th ed.). New York: Appleton-Century-Crofts, 1980.

Hudak, C.M., Lohr, T., and Gallo, B. *Critical care nursing.* Philadelphia: J.B. Lippincott, 1982.

Kempin, S. Disorders of hemostasis in malignancy. In A.D. Turnbull (Ed.), *Current problems in cancer* (vol. 4, no. 4.). Chicago: Year Book Medical Publishers, 1979, pp. 21-26.

Kinney, M.R., et al. *A.A.C.N.'s clinical reference for critical care nursing.* New York: McGraw-Hill, 1981.

Luckman, J., and Sorensen, K.C. *Medical-surgical nursing—A psychophysiologic approach* (2nd ed.). Philadelphia: W.B. Saunders, 1980.

Rothweiler, T.M. Coping with the complications of cancer. *RN*, **46**(9), 1983, 56–65.

Wroblewski, S.S., and Wroblewski, S.H. Caring for the patient with chemotherapy-induced thrombocytopenia. *American Journal of Nursing*, **81**(4), 1981, 746–749.

Zucker, M.B. The functioning of blood platelets. *Scientific American*, **242**(6), 1980, 86–103.

11. Disseminated Intravascular Coagulation

Disseminated intravascular coagulation (DIC), also called defibrination syndrome, consumptive coagulopathy, and diffuse intravascular clotting, is an abnormal activation of the clotting mechanism caused by the disease process of cancer and certain chemotherapeutic drugs. The hemorrhagic form of DIC is seen in 10% of all clients with cancer. The normal coagulation process consists of the following events.

1. Vascular injury → release of tissue thromboplastin
2. Thromboplastin + 7 factors + prothrombin → thrombin
3. Thrombin + fibrinogen → fibrin
4. Fibrin + platelets → clot formation
5. Fibrinolysin → clot degradation

Cancer cells can produce abnormal amounts of tissue thromboplastin when they adhere to vascular endothelium to establish their blood supply, causing a rapid "using up" or consumption of the clotting factors and platelets. Bleeding occurs when the thrombin activity is abnormally excessive, and abnormal coagulation occurs when the fibrinolysis activity is excessive. When microthrombi form in the capillaries, microinfarctions cause ischemia and cellular necrosis of major organs. DIC can be exogenous or endogenous. Exogenous DIC is usually triggered by transfusion reactions, septicemia, or release of thrombin or thromboplastin from cancer cells. Endogenous DIC results from a slow, continuous production of thromboplastin with cellular necrosis. Thrombocytopenia, decreased serum fibrinogen, and increased prothrombin time are characteristic and diagnostic of DIC.

Vincristine, methotrexate, 6-mercaptopurine, prednisone, and L-asparaginase are possible chemotherapeutic agents that cause DIC. Corresponding cancers include acute promyelocytic leukemia, lung, lymphoma, gallbladder, stomach, colon, breast, ovary, melanoma, pancreas, and prostate. Additional causes include infection, surgery, shock, incompatible blood transfusions, collagen vascular diseases, aortic aneurysms, and amyloidosis (Chapter 33).

ASSESSMENT DATA

- Thrombocytopenia
- Increased prothrombin time and fibrinogen degradation products (FDP)
- Decreased serum fibrinogen
- Bleeding or thrombosis of

    Skin—ecchymose, purpura, petechiae, acral cyanosis (ecchymose over digits that can progress to gangrene)

    Mucous membranes—epistaxis, conjunctiva

    GI tract—frank or occult blood in stools, hematemesis, absent or high pitch bowel sounds

    GU tract—hematuria, menorrhagia, metrorrhagia, oliguria, anuria, azotemia, elevated BUN, or creatinine

    Lungs—hemoptysis, dyspnea, cyanosis, hypoxia

    CNS—change in LOC, restlessness

    Retina—blurred or decrease in vision

    Joints—pain or stiffness

- Shock symptoms with hemorrhage—hypotension, tachycardia; cold, pale, moist skin
- Decrease hemoglobin and hematocrit
- Thrombophlebitis

NURSING DIAGNOSES

Potential alteration in cardiac output, decreased, related to abnormal blood clotting mechanism(s), resulting in bleeding or coagulation.

Alterations in tissue perfusion, related to ischemia and cellular necrosis, resulting from microthrombi forming microinfarctions.

RATIONALE

Blood volume is decreased as a result of increased amounts of tissue thromboplastin, increased thrombin activity, and/or increased fibrinolysis activity.

Interruption of blood flow to an organ or structure results in tissue hypoxia and cellular death.

NURSING INTERVENTIONS

Monitoring–Independent

1. Blood pressure, heart rate, respirations q 1 hr during acute phase, q 2 hr after stabilization. Do not overinflate cuff.

2. Oral temperature q 4 hr (fever destroys platelets).
3. Hourly I and O and calculate I/O ratio for fluid balance q 8 and 24 hr.
4. Assess skin for color, temperature, moisture, and discolorations q 4 to 8 hr.
5. Assess leg calf bilaterally for pain, tenderness, and swelling q 8 hr. Do NOT assess for Homan sign. (Homan sign maneuver can dislodge thrombi and cause emboli.)
6. Auscultate heart sounds at 4 valvular sites q 4 to 8 hr and record onset of gallop.
7. Auscultate lung sounds in all fields, symmetry of chest expansion, and use of accessory breathing muscles q 4 to 8 hr and record onset of rales, rhonchi, or wheeze.
8. Inspect all sputum for color, amount, and consistency.
9. Assess for chest pain and headache q 8 hr.
10. Urine specific gravity q 4 to 8 hr if urinary output becomes progressively decreased.
11. Auscultate bowel sounds and assess abdomen for rebound tenderness, firmness, and distention q 4 to 8 hr.
12. Hemocult all stools and emesis.
13. Assess LOC q 4 to 8 hr or with each contact if DIC impending and record changes in awareness, orientation, and behavior.
14. Assess all orifices, venipuncture sites, surgical incisions, and surgical drain sites for bleeding or oozing q 4 to 8 hr.
15. Assess major joints for pain or stiffness during ROME.
16. Assess peripheral pulses for bilateral quality q 8 hr.
17. Assess IV site for redness, swelling, and pain q 4 to 8 hr.

Monitoring–Interdependent

1. Assess laboratory data when available and compare to previous and normal values and those indicating DIC or complications of DIC:

	NORMS	DIC
Platelet count	130,000 to 370,000/mm^3	<130,000
Prothrombin time	Control plus 4 sec	Prolonged
Partial thromboplastin time	Control plus 10 sec	Prolonged
Fibrinogen	200 to 500 mg/dl	Decreased
Fibrinogen degradation products	<12 mg/ml	>12 mg/ml
Hemoglobin	13.0 to 18.0 g/dl males	Decreased
	12.0 to 16.0 g/dl females	Decreased
Hematocrit	45 to 52% males	Decreased
	37 to 48% females	Decreased

Lee–White clotting time	6 to 17 min	Prolonged
ABGs: pH	7.35 to 7.45	Decreased
(adult) Pco_2	35 to 45 torr	Increased
Po_2	75 to 100 torr	Decreased
HCO_3	24 to 30 mEq/L	Same or Increased
O_2 saturation	95 to 100%	Decreased
BE	±2 mEq/L	Positive
CO_2 content	24 to 30 mEq/L	Increased

These abnormal values would reflect respiratory acidosis if pulmonary thromboembolism or shock lung developed as a complication of DIC.

2. Question use of aspirin, Darvon, Foley catheters, suppositories, unnecessary or frequent IM injections, and rectal temperatures.
3. Assess for adverse reactions during blood transfusions. Discontinue transfusion if dyspnea, hematuria, fever, chills, or lumbar pain develops indicating hemolytic reaction.

Change–Independent

1. Bedrest and minimize activity with platelet count of less than 50,000 mm³.
2. Apply direct pressure to all venipuncture sites for 10 min or until bleeding stops.
3. Force fluids to 120 ml q 1 hr while awake if applicable.
4. File fingernails to shortest length and use soft brush to clean qd.
5. Coordinate all laboratory work so that venipunctures are minimized.
6. Use smallest gauge needles appropriate to IV infusions and parenteral injections.
7. Turn, cough, deep breathe q 2 hr.
8. Oral and teeth care using sponge tip applicators and half-strength H_2O_2 q 4 to 8 hr and rinse thoroughly. Once a day, use a mixture of H_2O_2 and baking soda to neutralize acid and remove plaque.
9. Light massage using nonastringent lotions to all bony prominences q 4 hr.
10. Bathe, without soap, using commercially prepared bath emollients qd.
11. Make frequent physical and visual contact with client during acute phase stating time of return before leaving.
12. Reorient time, place, and reason for hospitalization with each contact if client confused or disoriented.
13. Eliminate all environmental hazards to safety. Keep side rails up and pad if client restless or disoriented; put bed in low position, and place call light and personal articles within easy reach.
14. Passive ROME to all major joints q 4 hr if tolerated.
15. Explain condition and progress to client and family with each contact.

Assist them to ask questions and express concerns of the present and future.

16. Include family members in plan of care and allow them to participate, if mutually beneficial.

17. Teach client to (if applicable):
    Eliminate nose trauma from blowing or picking
    Eliminate valsalva maneuver by consciously preventing straining during defecation or holding breath when changing position.
    Eliminate use of dental floss, toothpicks, tampons.

17. Before all procedures, explain purpose and technique in understandable terms.

Change–Interdependent

1. D5W at KVO or as prescribed by physician.

2. Notify physician if:
    Platelet count less than 100,000 and prothrombin time and partial thromboplastin time prolonged
    Hemoglobin less than 10 g/dl
    Hematocrit less than 35%
    Abnormal ABGs, especially Po_2 less than 75 torr
    BP systolic 90 torr or less
    Active, profuse bleeding occurs from any site or any occurrence of signs and symptoms of multisystem involvement or complications

3. Anticipate the physician to prescribe:
    Platelet transfusion if thrombocyte count less than 50,000 mm^3
    Heparin: continuous IV infusion, 10 to 15 units/kg to decrease thrombin activity and inhibit activity of thromboplastic substance. (This is very controversial.)
    Antithrombin III concentrate: experimental therapy
    EACA (epsilon aminocaproic acid): 5 g slow IV push initial dose, then 2 g q 1 to 2 hr x 24 hr, an antifibrinolytic agent. Side effects include: hypokalemia, hypotension, arrhythmias, and intravascular coagulation.
    Antacids and stool softeners to decrease GI irritation
    Pack nose with gauze soaked with adrenalin 1:10,000 to stop epistaxis.
    Ice lavage to stop bleeding in upper GI tract
    Ice enema to stop bleeding in lower GI tract

BIBLIOGRAPHY

Bell, W.R. Disseminated intravascular coagulation. *The Johns Hopkins Medical Journal*, **146**(6), 1980, 289–299.

Bick, R.L. Disseminated intravascular coagulation and related syndromes: Etiology, pathophysiology, diagnosis, and management. *American Journal of Hematology,* **5,** 1978, 265-282.

Caprini, J.A., and Sener, S.F. Altered coagulability in cancer patients. *CA-A Cancer Journal for Clinicians,* **32**(3), 1982, 162-172.

Corbett, J.V. *Laboratory tests in nursing practice.* Norwalk, Connecticut: Appleton-Century-Crofts, 1982.

Gordon, M. *Manual of nursing diagnosis.* New York: McGraw-Hill, 1982.

Hasegawa, D.K., and Bloomfield, C.D. Thrombotic and hemorrhagic manifestations of malignancy. In J. Yarbro and R. Bornstein (Eds.), *Oncologic emergencies.* New York: Grune and Stratton, 1981, pp. 141-196.

Hudak, C.M., Lohr, T., and Gallo, B. *Critical care nursing.* Philadelphia: J.B. Lippincott, 1982.

Johanson, B.C., et al. *Standards for critical care.* St. Louis: C.V. Mosby, 1981.

Kinney, M.R., et al. *A.A.C.N.'s clinical reference for critical care nursing.* New York: McGraw-Hill, 1981.

Kirchner, C.W., and Reheis, C.E. Two serious complications of neoplasia: Sepsis and disseminated intravascular coagulation. *Nursing Clinics of North America,* **17**(4), 1982, 595-606.

Luckmann, J., and Sorensen, K.C. *Medical-surgical nursing—A psychophysiologic approach* (2nd ed.). Philadelphia: W.B. Saunders, 1980.

McGillick, K. DIC: The deadly paradox. *RN,* **45**(8), 1982, 41-43.

Rothweiler, T.M. Coping with the complications of cancer. *RN,* **46**(9), 1983, 56-65.

Timms, J. Disseminated intravascular coagulation as an oncologic emergency. Paper presented at the *Second Oncology Nursing Seminar, Clemson University,* College of Nursing, Clemson, South Carolina, April 1981.

Yasko, J.M., and Schafer, S.L. Disseminated intravascular coagulation. In *Guidelines for cancer care—Symptom management.* Joyce M. Yasko (Ed.), Virginia: Reston, 1983, pp. 324-329.

Zucker, M.B. The functioning of blood platelets. *Scientific American,* **242**(6), 1980, 86-103.

12. Endogenous Hemorrhagic Gastritis

DEFINITION AND CAUSATIVE FACTORS

Endogenous hemorrhagic gastritis resulting in massive bleeding develops from gastric malignancies, from antineoplastic drug therapy, and from secondary factors, such as stress ulcers and frequent administration of pain medications that irritate the gastric mucosa. Gastric malignancies cause erosion of major arterial vessels after infiltrating the gastric wall or by direct extension involving adjacent structures. Chemotherapeutic agents target all rapidly growing cells, including the endothelial cells of the gastric mucosa, stripping the stomach of its protective mucosal barrier against acid. All critically ill clients will develop gastric erosions to some degree, but the client with cancer has a greater risk when antineoplastic drugs are added to the therapeutic regimen. Gastrointestinal bleeding has a mortality rate of 45%, and the problem is aggravated by sepsis, thrombocytopenia, uremia, and liver involvement. Diagnosis is confirmed by an upper GI series or endoscopy. The color of the blood is a significant parameter of assessment data (Table 12-1).

Corresponding cancers include gastric carcinoid tumors, gastric lymphomas, melanoma, leukemia, and cancers of the genitourinary tract, breast, and lung. Ulcers, sepsis, and anticoagulants are additional causes.

ASSESSMENT DATA

- Identified site of bleeding demonstrated by x-ray or endoscopy
- Decreased hemoglobin, hematocrit
- Thrombocytopenia
- Decreased prothrombin time and PTT
- Hematemesis, melena

- History of chemotherapy, stress ulcers, anticoagulants, uremia, hepatic disease
- Positive cultures indicating sepsis
- Decreased blood pressure
- Tachycardia
- Pallor
- Restlessness
- Tachypnea
- Vomiting
- Weakness
- Abdominal distention
- Increased BUN (an elevated BUN of 40 mg/dl with a normal creatinine indicates bleeding in the upper GI tract of 1000 ml or more).

NURSING DIAGNOSES

Fluid volume deficit, related to acute or chronic blood loss, resulting from mucosal erosion.

Associated Nursing Diagnoses

1. Alteration in nutrition, less than body requirements, related to the inability of the GI tract to absorb nutrients resulting in nutritional deficiencies.

RATIONALE

Over two-thirds of intestinal blood flow is to the mucosa.

Absorptive area of the mucosa is decreased due to the destruction of the folds of kerkring, villi, and microvilli.

NURSING INTERVENTIONS

Monitoring–Independent

1. BP, heart rate, respirations q 15 to 30 min with bleeding episode, q 1 to 2 hr with onset of symptoms other than active bleeding.
2. Hemocult all stools and vomitus, and record.
3. Assess LOC q 8 hr and record changes in awareness, orientation, and behavior.
4. Auscultate bowel sounds in 4 quadrants q 8 hr and record onset and location of changes in pitch and frequency.

TABLE 12-1. ACUTE GASTROINTESTINAL
BLEEDING: SIGNIFICANCE OF COLOR OF BLOOD

Color	Significance
Bright red blood	Fresh blood; massive bleeding
Bright red vomitus	Fresh blood from duodenum or stomach
Dark-red or coffee-ground vomitus	Old blood-perhaps several hours; from duodenum or stomach

NOTE: Gastric acid turns bright-red blood (red hemoglobin) to dark-red (brown hematin). The brighter the blood, generally, the shorter the time spent in contact with gastric acid.

Tarry stools	Only 60 ml of blood in the GI tract is necessary to cause this symptom—usually from duodenal rather than gastric ulcers. Most commonly associated with upper GI bleeding, although can occur in lower GI bleeding.
With diarrhea	Bleeding is above the duodenojejunal junction (ligament of Treitz)
Without diarrhea	Bleeding is above the midtransverse colon
Passing of bright red blood which may coat surface of stool	Seen with lower GI bleeding—that is, lower sigmoid and rectum
Maroon-colored blood with diarrhea	Bleeding is located above midtransverse colon
Bright red blood with stool	Bleeding is located below midtransverse colon
Blood and pus with stool	Inflammatory disease (ulcerative colitis)
Dark-red or currant-jelly color	Bleeding is located at Meckel's diverticulum

Source: Fletcher, B. *Quick Reference to Critical Care*. Philadelphia: J.B. Lippincott, 1983, p. 267, with permission.

5. Assess client for abdominal pain with each contact and describe:
    Location
    Radiation
    Duration
    Intensity
    Aggravating and alleviating factors
6. Palpate abdomen for rigidity, distention, general and rebound tenderness q 4 to 8 hr. Measure abdominal girth utilizing predetermined marks q 2 hr (if applicable).
7. Hourly I and O, calculate I/O ratio for fluid balance q 8 and 24 hr.
8. Weigh q AM before breakfast and compare to previous measurements.
9. Temperature q 4 hr.
10. Assess skin color, temperature, moisture, and discoloration q 4 to 8 hr.

11. Assess heart sounds in 4 valvular locations q 8 hr and record changes in rate and rhythm.

12. Palpate peripheral pulses for bilateral quality q 8 hr.

13. Assess client for nausea and vomiting with each contact.

14. Determine skin turgor, muscle firmness, and presence of dependent edema q 8 hr.

15. Assess objective and subjective indications of restlessness or fatigue with each client contact.

16. Assess IV site or TPN site for pain, redness or swelling q 2 hr.

Monitoring–Interdependent

1. Assess results of laboratory data when available and compare to previous and normal values.

   CBC   Hemoglobin: 13.0 to 18.0 g/dl males

   　　　　　　　　　12.0 to 16.0 g/dl females

   　　　　Hematocrit: 45 to 52% males

   　　　　　　　　37 to 48% females

   　　　　RBC: 4.6 to 6.2 $\times$ 10^6/mm^3 males

   　　　　　　　4.2 to 5.4 $\times$ 10^6/mm^3 females

   　　　　MCH: 27 to 32 pg

   　　　　MCHC: 32 to 36%

   　　　　MCV: 80 to 94 cu microns

   　　　　Platelets: 130,000 to 370,000 mm^3

   　　　　WBC: 4,500 to 11,500/mm^3

   Prothrombin Time: control + 4 sec

   Partial Thromboplastin Time: control + 10 sec

   Coagulation Time (Lee–White): 6 to 17 min

   Serum Sodium: 135 to 145 mEq/L

   Serum Potassium: 3.5 to 5.0 mEq/L

   Serum Chloride: 100 to 106 mEq/L

   Serum Calcium: 8.5 to 10.5 mg/dl

   Serum Magnesium: 1.5 to 2.0 mEq/L

   Serum Phosphorus: 3.0 to 4.5 mg/dl

   Blood Proteins: 6.0 to 8.4 g/dl

   Albumin: 3.5 to 5.5 g/dl

   BUN: 8 to 25 mg/dl

   Creatinine: 0.6 to 1.5 mg/dl

   Blood Sugar: 70 to 100 mg/dl

   Blood Cultures: positive for sepsis

2. Urine sugar and acetone q 6 hr if TPN prescribed and solution contains more than 5% dextrose.

3. Assess client for blood transfusion reaction q 15 min ×4 then q 1 hr (if applicable).
   Fever, chills
   Hives, itching
   Dyspnea, wheezing
   Lumbar, chest pain
   Oliguria, hematuria
   Nausea
   Paresthesia

Change-Independent

1. Maintain bedrest with hemoglobin 10 g/dl or less, or when acute bleeding episode occurs.
2. Mouth care q 4 hr and after each vomiting episode using $\frac{1}{2}$ strength H_2O_2 and a soft toothbrush. Once a day, clean teeth with a paste of H_2O_2 and baking soda to neutralize oral acid and remove plaque.
3. Perirectal skin care after each diarrheal episode and apply protective agent.
4. Offer 120 ml of clear liquids q 2 hr if tolerated and po fluids not restricted.
5. Apply ice collar to neck with onset of nausea.
6. Bathe using commercially prepared bath emollient.
7. Back care q 4 hr using mild friction with lotion to all bony prominences.
8. Turn, cough, deep breathe q 2 hr while on bedrest.
9. Position on side with persistent vomiting.
10. Passive ROME to all major joints q 4 hr while on bedrest.
11. Institute all safety measures with onset of weakness by elevating side rails and pad if client becomes restless, and arranging call light and personal articles within easy reach.
12. O_2 at 2 L/min by nasal cannula if SOB occurs with decreased hemoglobin.
13. Maintain frequent physical and visual contact with client during acute bleeding episodes stating time of return before leaving.
14. Reorient to time, place, and reason for hospitalization with each contact if client confused or disoriented.
15. Explain purpose and techniques of all procedures in understandable terms.
16. Explain condition and progress to client and family with each contact. Assist them to ask questions and express concerns of the present and the future.

17. Include family members in plan of care and allow them to participate, if mutually beneficial.

Change–Interdependent

1. Discontinue blood transfusion if fever, itching, chills, dyspnea, rales, chest tightness, paresthesia, lumbar pain, and tachypnea occurs.
2. Slow blood transfusion rate if chills, hives, and mild wheezing occur.
3. Administer antiemetic and analgesic medications and assess effect in 10 to 20 min.
4. Notify physician if:
    Hematemesis or melena occur
    Blood transfusion reactions occur
    Systolic blood pressure 90 torr or less
    Onset of abnormal bowel sounds with abdominal rigidity and rebound tenderness occur
    BUN greater than 25 mg/dl with normal creatinine
    Serum potassium greater than 6 mEq/L
    Serum calcium less than 8.0 mg/dl
    Blood sugar less than 60 mg/dl or greater than 350
    Hemoglobin less than 10 g/dl
    Hematocrit less than 30%
    Platelet count less than 100,000 mm^3
    Prothrombin time greater than control + 4 sec
    Partial thromboplastin time greater than control + 10 sec
    Blood cultures positive indicating sepsis
5. Anticipate physician to prescribe:
    TPN with persistent vomiting or diarrhea greater than 3 days
    Blood transfusions with hemoglobin less than 10 g/dl or hematocrit less than 30%
    NG tube insertion and intermittent or continuous iced saline irrigation until clear (Table 12-2)
    Levophed (2 amps/1000 ml saline) by NG tube to effect vasoconstriction
    Topical thrombin (5000 units in 5 ml saline) by NG tube. Thrombin, along with fibrinogen, clots the bleeding.
    Vitamin K to facilitate blood clotting.
Pitressin IV to decrease portal hypertension and flow of blood to the stomach. It can cause hypertension and decreased urinary output as side effects.
Tagamet IV to reduce gastric hyperacidity

TABLE 12-2. GASTRIC LAVAGE
FOR PATIENT WITH ACUTE GI BLEEDING

NOTE: Check for tube placement prior to instillation of solution.

ICED SALINE METHOD

1. Instill 200 ml to 300 ml of iced saline into the stomach, using a continuous infusion system.
2. Clamp the tube to the irrigating solution.
3. Allow the solution to remain in the stomach for 2 to 3 min to promote vasoconstriction.
4. Unclamp drainage tube and siphon out solution by manual aspiration, using a 50-ml syringe or gravity drainage into collection bottle.
5. Using a 50-ml irrigating syringe, manually irrigate the tube frequently to dislodge blood clots regardless of the method used for solution drainage.
6. Repeat the above procedure, as specified by the physician, until the returns are clear or faint pink.

NOTES:

- Do not use iced water as the irrigating solution because this may cause electrolyte depletion.
- Iced saline may cause an increase in circulating volume in susceptible patients due to absorption of sodium chloride. Monitor patient closely for signs of pulmonary edema and congestive heart failure.

ICED SALINE WITH LEVOPHED METHOD

1. Add 2 to 4 ampules of Levophed (levarterenol) to 1000 ml of normal saline (irrigating solution).
   Levophed causes vasoconstriction. Systemic effects are prevented by its absorption from the stomach into the portal system and subsequent transport to the liver, where drug metabolism occurs.
2. Follow procedure for irrigating with iced saline.

Source: Fletcher, B. *Quick Reference to Critical Care*. Philadelphia: J.B. Lippincott, 1983, p. 269, with permission.

Progression to oral diet from clear liquids to liquids, to soft, bland, 6 small meals as prescribed. (If client acidotic from severe, prolonged undernourishment omit citrus fruit juices.)

BIBLIOGRAPHY

Barber, J., Stokes, L., and Billings, D. *Adult and child care* (2nd ed.). St. Louis: C.V. Mosby, 1977.

Barber, J.M., and Budassi, S.A. *Manual of emergency care—Practices and procedures*. St. Louis: C.V. Mosby, 1979.

Burkhart, C. Upper GI hemorrhage: The clinical picture. *American Journal of Nursing*, 1981, 1817–1820.

Corbett, J.V. *Laboratory tests in nursing practice*. Norwalk, Connecticut: Appleton-Century-Crofts, 1982.

Gordon, M. *Manual of nursing diagnosis*. New York: McGraw-Hill, 1982.

Harvey, A.M., Johns, R.J., McKusick, V.A., Owens, A.H., Jr., and Ross, R.S. *The principles and practice of medicine* (20th ed.). New York: Appleton-Century-Crofts, 1980.

Horton, J., and Hill, G.J. *Clinical oncology*. Philadelphia: W.B. Saunders, 1977.

Hudak, C.M., Lohr, T., and Gallo, B. *Critical care nursing*. Philadelphia: J.B. Lippincott, 1982.

Jeejeebhoy, K. A critical type of upper GI bleeding. *Emergency Medicine*, 14(5), 1982, 47–57.

Johanson, B.C., et al. *Standards for critical care*. St. Louis: C.V. Mosby, 1981.

Lamphier, T.A., and Lamphier, R.A. Upper GI hemorrhage: Emergency evaluation and management. *American Journal of Nursing*, 81(10), 1981, 1814–1817.

Luckman, J., and Sorensen, K.C. *Medical-surgical nursing—A psychophysiologic approach* (2nd ed.). Philadelphia. W.B. Saunders, 1980.

Riepe, S.P. Acute lower gastrointestinal bleeding. *Critical Care Quarterly*, 5(2), 1982, 29–32.

13. Superior Vena Cava Syndrome

DEFINITION AND CAUSATIVE FACTORS

Superior vena cava syndrome (SVCS) occurs when the superior vena cava (SVC) is occluded by external pressure, invaded by a neoplasm, or obstructed by a large intraluminal thrombosis causing an impairment in venous return from the head and upper extremities. Venous hypertension, delayed circulation time, and venous dilatation of collateral venous circulation are the bases of the physical manifestations. The SVC is susceptible to obstruction because it is located in a tight compartment surrounded by ribs, sternum, and vertebrae. The onset and severity of SVCS depends on the size and location of the obstruction and the success or failure of collateral circulation to maintain venous flow (Figure 13-1). Compression of adjacent structures also occur—trachea, bronchial nerves, major blood vessels, and spinal cord. Pleural effusion is a common complication. Obstruction due to a thrombotic occlusion with tumor compression should be suspected if the symptoms do not abate with radiation and/or chemotherapy.

Corresponding cancers include oat cell carcinoma of the lung, bronchogenic, non-Hodgkin lymphoma, breast, Kaposi sarcoma, and testicular metastasis. Aortic aneurysm, benign tumors, histoplasmosis, tuberculosis, and postradiation are additional causes.

ASSESSMENT DATA

- Facial swelling upon rising in AM
- Periorbital edema
- Red conjunctivitis in AM
- Edema arms, hands, neck, trunk
- Funduscopic exam—dilatated retinal veins and conjunctival edema

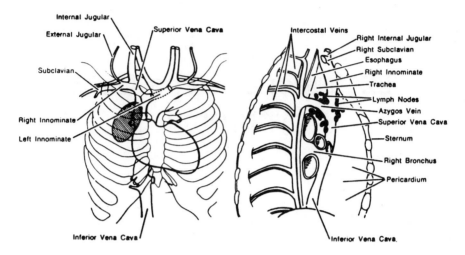

Figure 13-1. Schematic representation of the frontal (*left*) and saggital (*right*) sections of the thorax showing the relationship of the azygos vein the superior vena cava (SVC), coalescence of innominates to form the SVC at the right second rib, and the encasement of the SVC by nodal structures. Shaded area indicates classical site of obstruction. Source: DeVita, et al. (Eds.). Cancer, principles, practice of oncology. Philadelphia, J.B. Lippincott, 1982, with permission.

- Distended veins of the neck and/or chest
- Shortness of breath
- Cyanosis
- Chest pain
- Dysphagia
- Frequent coughing
- Headache
- Decreased LOC
- Decreased visual acuity
- Impaired short- or long-term memory
- Horner syndrome (one-sided eyelid drooping, pupil constriction, conjunctivitis, absence of sweat).
- Vocal cord paralysis
- Tachycardia
- Tachypnea
- Chest x-ray demonstrating mediastinal mass

NURSING DIAGNOSES	RATIONALE
Alteration in cardiac output, decreased, related to SVC occlusion, resulting in impaired venous return to the heart and decreased cardiac output.	*Venous hypertension results in areas normally drained by the SVC which empties into the right atrium of the heart.*

Associated Nursing Diagnoses

1. Ineffective breathing pattern, related to the compression of respiratory structures and a decrease in circulating blood volume, resulting in hypoxia.

   Inadequate oxygenation resulting from obstruction and decreased circulating time.

2. Sensory deficit, uncompensated, related to cerebral venous hypertension, resulting in increased intracranial pressure and loss of cerebral function of vision and altered level of consciousness.

   Level of consciousness and vision are impaired by oxygen deprivation.

3. Cognitive impairment, related to cerebral hypertension, resulting in loss of cerebral function for memory, judgment, and reasoning.

   Occlusion or obstruction of the the SVC vessel enhances cerebral hypertension.

NURSING INTERVENTIONS

Monitoring–Independent

1. BP, heart rate, and respirations every 5 to 15 min if acute condition, every 1 hr with onset of symptoms.
2. Assess degree of facial and periorbital edema, and distended superficial chest veins, and record changes every 4 to 8 hr. Periorbital edema most noticeable upon rising in the AM.
3. Assess for pulsus alternans q 4 hr (unpalpable pulse during inspiration).
4. Assess skin color, temperature, moisture every 4 to 8 hr.
5. Assess LOC q 4 to 8 hr and record changes in awareness, orientation, and behavior.

6. Hourly urinary outputs; calculate I/O ratio for fluid balance every 8 and 24 hr.

7. Palpate peripheral pulses for bilateral quality q 8 hr.

8. Assess neck vein distention in cm q 4 to 8 hr.

9. Assess tissue perfusion by blanching nail test q 8 hr.

10. Auscultate breath sounds in all lung fields, symmetry of chest expansion, and use of accessory muscles q 4 to 8 hr, and record onset of adventitious sounds.

11. Assess for dyspnea and respiratory distress with each client contact.

12. Assess ability to swallow with all po fluids, foods, or medication.

13. Assess client's voice quality and record changes in pitch, clarity, and hoarseness with each client contact.

14. Assess IV site for pain, redness, swelling q 8 hr.

15. Assess for pain in chest and for headache with each client contact.

Monitoring–Interdependent

1. Assess CVP q 2 hr or as prescribed and compare to previous and normal measurements: 4 to 8 mm H_2O.

2. Assess laboratory data when available and compare to previous and normal values.

    ABGs: pH: 7.35 to 7.45
    Po_2: 75 to 100 torr
    Pco_2: 35 to 45 torr
    HCO_3: 24 to 30 mEq/L
    O_2 Saturation: 95 to 100%
    BE: ± 2 mEq/L
    CO_2 Content: 24 to 30 mEq/L

    Serum Sodium: 135 to 145 mEq/L
    Serum Potassium: 3.5 to 5.0 mEq/L
    Serum Chloride: 100 to 106 mEq/L
    Serum Calcium: 8.5 to 10.5 mg/dl
    BUN: 8 to 25 mg/dl
    Creatinine: 0.6 to 1.5 mg/dl
    CBC: Hemoglobin: 13.0 to 18.0 g/dl males
    12.0 to 16.0 g/dl females
    Hematocrit: 45 to 52% males
    37 to 48% females
    RBC: 4.6 to 6.2 × 10^6/mm^3 males
    4.2 to 5.4 × 10^6/mm^3 females
    WBC: 4,500 to 11,500/mm^3
    MCH: 27 to 32 pg

MCHC: 32 to 36%
MCV: 80 to 94 microns
Prothrombin Time: control + 4 sec
Partial Thromboplastin Time: control + 10 sec
Lee-White Clotting Time: 6 to 17 min

3. Assess results of chest x-ray, bronchoscopy, mediastinoscopy when available.

Change–Independent

1. Apply O_2 by nasal cannula at 2 L/min or as prescribed.
2. Maintain bedrest and elevate HOB to 60°.
3. Minimize activity during hypovolemic and dyspneic episodes.
4. Turn side to back to side in sitting position and deep breathe q 2 hr.
5. Massage all bony prominences q 4 hr with lotion while on bedrest.
6. Discontinue po intake with indication of dysphagia.
7. Mouth care using soft toothbrush and mouth wash q 4 hr. Once a day, clean teeth with a paste of H_2O_2 and baking soda to neutralize oral acid and remove plaque.
8. Passive ROME to all extremities q 4 hr except during critical phases.
9. Before all procedures, explain purpose and technique in understandable terms.
10. Reorient to time, place, reason for hospitalization if client confused or disoriented.
11. Eliminate all environmental safety hazards. Keep side rails up and pad if client restless and disoriented. Place call light and personal articles within easy reach.
12. Explain condition and progress to client and family with each contact. Assist them to ask questions and express concerns of the present and the future.
13. Include family members in plan of care and allow them to participate, if mutually beneficial.
14. Maintain frequent physical and visual contact with client during critical phases stating time of return before leaving.

Change–Interdependent

1. D5W at KVO or as prescribed by physican.
2. Medicate appropriately for pain and anxiety as prescribed and assess effect in 10 to 20 min.
3. Irrigate NG tube with 10 to 20 ml saline q 4 hr after assessing correct placement, *or*

4. Consult with physician concerning need for soft, small, frequent meal diet if swallowing function adequate.

5. Notify physician if:
   Onset of facial, neck, or trunk edema occurs
   Systolic BP less than 90 torr
   Dyspnea, respiratory distress, dysphagia, aphasia occurs
   Urinary output 30 ml/hr or less
   Changes in LOC or vomiting occurs with facial and neck edema
   Po_2 less than 75 torr

6. Anticipate physician to prescribe:
   Chemotherapy
   Radiation therapy—4000 to 6000 rads over 5 to 7 wk for bronchogenic carcinoma and 2000 to 4000 rads for malignant lymphoma
   Combination chemoradiotherapy
   Anticoagulants to minimize or prevent clot formation due to venous statis in the SVC
   Diuretics to relieve edema
   Steroids to reduce obstruction by decreasing inflammation caused by tumor invasion or compression

BIBLIOGRAPHY

Adria Laboratories, Inc. Chemotherapy of cancer. Part VI. How to handle special oncologic problems. Reprinted from *Drug Therapy*, August 1980.

Carabell, S.C., and Goodman, R.L. Superior vena caval syndrome. In V.T. DeVita, S. Hellman, and S.A. Rosenberg (Eds.), *Cancer, principles and practice of oncology.* Philadelphia: J.B. Lippincott, 1982, pp. 1582–1586.

Corbett, J.V. *Laboratory tests in nursing practice.* Norwalk, Connecticut: Appleton-Century-Crofts, 1982.

Davenport, D., et al. Response of superior vena cava syndrome to radiation therapy. *Cancer,* 38(4), 1976, 1577–1580.

Donoghue, M. Superior vena caval syndrome. In J.M. Yasko(Ed.), *Guidelines for cancer care—Symptom management.* Virginia: Reston, 1983, pp. 358–361.

Forman, J.W., and Unger, K. Unilateral superior vena caval syndrome. *Thorax,* **35,** 1980, 314–315.

Gettys, V.R. Oncologic emergencies: Superior vena cava syndrome. Paper presented at the *Second Oncology Nursing Seminar, Clemson University,* College of Nursing, Clemson, South Carolina, April 1981.

Gordon, M. *Manual of nursing diagnosis.* New York: McGraw-Hill, 1982.

Kane, R.C., et al. Superior vena caval obstruction due to small-cell anaplastic lung carcinoma: Response to chemotherapy. *JAMA,* **235,** 1976, 1717–1718.

Lockich, J.J., and Goodman, R. Superior vena cava syndrome. *JAMA,* **231,** 1976, 58–61.

Matthews, J.I., et al. Superior vena cava syndrome. *American Review of Respiratory Diseases*, 114(4), 1979, 683–684 (letter).

Nessenblatt, M.J. Oncologic emergencies. *American Family Physician*, 20(2), 1979, 104–114.

Nogeiere, C., et al. Long survival in patients with bronchogenic carcinoma complicated by superior vena caval obstruction. *Chest*, 75(3), 1979, 325–328.

Percarpio, B., and Gray, S. Prolonged survival following the superior vena cava syndrome. *Chest*, 75(5), 1979, 639–640.

Perez, C.A., et al. Management of superior vena cava syndrome. *Seminars in Oncology*, 5, 1978, 123–134.

Phipps, W.J., et al. *Medical-surgical nursing: Concepts and clinical practice.* St. Louis: C.V. Mosby, 1979.

Polackwich, R.J., and Straus, M.J. Superior vena caval syndrome. In M.J. Straus (Ed.), *Lung cancer: Clinical diagnosis and treatment.* New York: Grune and Stratton, 1977.

Sahn, S.A. Superior vena caval syndrome. In S.A. Sahn (Ed.), *Pulmonary emergencies.* New York: Churchill Livingstone, 1982, pp. 387–403.

Simpson, J.R., Perez, C.A., Presant, C.A., and Van Amburg, A.L. Superior vena cava syndrome. In J. Yarbro and R. Bornstein (Eds.), *Oncologic emergencies.* New York: Grune and Stratton, 1981, pp. 43–72.

Stolinsky, D.C. Emergencies in oncology—Current management. Superior vena cava obstruction. *Western Journal of Medicine*, 129, 1978, 169–170.

14. Neoplastic Pericardial Effusion and Tamponade

DEFINITION AND CAUSATIVE FACTORS

Cardiac tamponade occurs when the intrapericardial pressure increases sufficiently to restrict the expansion and movement of the left and right ventricles. It is caused by an accumulation of fluid into the pericardial space, tumor invasion of the mediastinum, and pericardial fibrosis and effusion from radiotherapy. As the left ventricular end diastolic volume and cardiac output decreases, pump failure and circulatory collapse ensues (cardiogenic shock). The critical stage develops when the onset of tamponade is rapid and compensatory tachycardia, peripheral vasoconstriction, and sodium–water retention cannot maintain the decreasing stroke volume. The onset of tamponade can be gradual or rapid, and the prognosis is poor if electrical alternans and pulsus paradoxus occurs. Because of the thoracic location of the tumor causing tamponade, other structures are also involved, especially the bronchi and lungs, producing respiratory manifestations.

Corresponding cancers include mesothelioma, sarcoma, leukemia, Hodgkin and non-Hodgkin lymphoma, melanoma, GI primaries, and metastatic tumors of the lung and breast. Radiation of 4,000 rads or more to the heart field, teratomas, fibromas, and angiomas are additional causes.

ASSESSMENT DATA

- Total electrical alternans—diagnostic of cardiac tamponade but usually a late sign
- Pulsus paradoxus greater than 10 mm Hg
- Narrowing pulse pressure
- Decreased systolic and increased diastolic BP
- Increased central venous pressure (CVP)
- Increased pulmonary artery systolic and diastolic pressure (PASP, PADP)

- Increased pulmonary capillary wedge pressure (PCWP)
- Decreased cardiac output
- Tachycardia
- Elevated "a" wave on RA pressure tracing during diastole
- Severe SOB
- Change in LOC
- Friction rub
- Muffled or distant heart sounds
- Murmur
- Decreased urinary output
- Pale, ashen, diaphoretic skin
- Anxiety and apprehension
- Knee–elbow sitting position
- Neck vein distention with HOB at 60°
- Hepatomegaly with hepatojugular reflux
- EKG changes—electrical alternans, decreased QRS voltage, T wave changes, elevated ST segment
- Chest x-ray—water bottle heart shadow

NURSING DIAGNOSES

Alteration in cardiac output, decreased, related to a reduced left ventricular end diastolic volume, cardiac output, and systolic blood pressure, resulting in pump failure and circulatory collapse.

RATIONALE

Cardiac output is severely decreased due to mechanical compression of the heart in diastole.

NURSING INTERVENTIONS

Monitoring–Independent

1. BP, heart rate, and respirations q 15 to 30 min if condition acute, q 1 hr with onset of symptoms, and record pulse pressure.
2. Assess for pulsus paradoxus with each BP measurement.
3. Assess cardiac monitor for a decrease in QRS voltage, electrical alternans (Fig. 14-1), elevated ST segment, T wave changes, and arrhythmias.
4. Auscultate heart sounds at 4 valvular sites q 2 to 4 hr and record quality

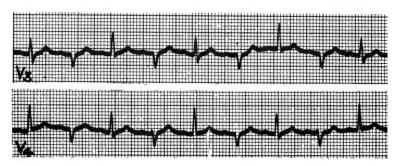

Figure 14-1. Electrical alternans. Note alternating direction of QRS complexes. Source: Marriott, H.J.L., 1977, with permission.

of S_1 and S_2 sounds and onset of friction rub—location and number of components.

5. Assess neck vein distention in cm with HOB at 60° q 2 to 4 hr.
6. Palpate peripheral pulses for bilateral quality q 4 to 8 hr.
7. Assess all dependent areas for edema q 4 to 8 hr.
8. Assess LOC q 4 to 8 hr and record changes in awareness, orientation, and behavior.
9. Assess skin color, temperature, and moisture q 4 to 8 hr.
10 Hourly I and O and calculate I/O ratio for fluid balance q 8 and 24 hr.
11. Auscultate all lung fields, symmetry of chest expansion, and use of accessory muscles q 4 to 8 hr and record onset of adventitious sounds.
12. Assess for dyspnea or respiratory distress with each client contact.
13. Oral temperature q 4 hr.
14. Assess IV site for redness, pain, swelling q 4 to 8 hr.

Monitoring–Interdependent

1. Assess hemodynamic pressure measurements after insertion of pulmonary artery flotation catheter (Swan–Ganz) and compare to previous and normal values (frequency depends on agency protocol or as prescribed by physician).

	NORMAL	TAMPONADE
PASP	20–30 torr	Increased
PADP	7–12 torr	Increased
PCWP	8–12 torr	Increased
Cardiac output	4–8 L/min	Decreased
Cardiac index	3.5 ± 0.7 L/min/m^2	Decreased
SVR	900–1200 units	Increased
CVP	0–5 torr	Increased

2. Assess laboratory data when available and compare to previous and normal values.

   ABGs pH: 7.35 to 7.45
   Po_2: 75 to 100 torr
   Pco_2: 35 to 45 torr
   HCO_3: 24 to 30 mEq/L
   O_2 Saturation: 95 to 100%
   BE: ± 2 mEq/L
   CO_2 Content: 24 to 30 mEq/L
   Serum Sodium: 135 to 145 mEq/L
   Serum Potassium: 3.5 to 5.0 mEq/L
   Serum Chloride: 100 to 106 mEq/L
   Serum Calcium: 8.5 to 10.5 mg/dl
   CBC Hemoglobin: 13.0 to 18.0 g/dl males
   12.0 to 16.0 g/dl females
   Hematocrit: 45 to 52% males
   37 to 48% females
   RBC: 4.6 to 6.2 × 10^6/mm^3 males
   4.2 to 5.4 × 10^6/mm^3 females
   MCH: 27 to 32 pg
   MCHC: 32 to 36%
   MCV: 80 to 94 cu microns
   Platelets: 130,000 to 370,000 mm^3
   WBC: 4,500 to 11,500/mm^3

3. Assess effects of unloading medications if prescribed.

   Nipride to decrease preload and afterload by vasodilatation

   Dopamine to increase velocity and force of contraction, ejection fraction, stroke volume, renal vasodilatation, and to decrease SVR (afterload)

   Lasix to diurese excess fluid volume once tamponade relieved, reduce afterload and venous return

   Digoxin to increase force of contraction once tamponade relieved

Change–Independent

1. Elevate HOB at 45 to 60° or position of greatest comfort.

2. Maintain on bedrest and minimize activity.

3. Apply humidified O_2 by nasal cannula at 2 L/min or as prescribed by physician.

4. Maintain client on NPO unless otherwise specified.

5. Mouth care using soft toothbrush and mouthwash or other oral antiseptic q 4 to 8 hr. Once a day, clean teeth with a mixture of H_2O_2 and baking soda to neutralize oral acid and remove plaque.

6. Turn, cough, deep breathe q 2 hr if tolerance permits.
7. Sponge bathe with tepid water after diaphoretic episodes when client's condition stabilizes.
8. Passive ROME to all major joints 3 times a day if tolerated.
9. Maintain frequent physical and visual contact with client during immediate life-threatening phase stating time of return before leaving.
10. Reorient to time, place, and reason for hospitalization with each contact if client confused or disoriented.
11. Before all procedures, explain purpose and technique in understandable terms.
12. Explain condition and progress to client and family with each contact. Assist them to ask questions and express concerns of the present and the future.
13. Eliminate all environmental hazards to safety. Keep side rails up and pad if client restless and disoriented. Place call bell within easy reach.

Change–Interdependent

1. D5W at KVO or as prescribed by physician.
2. Medicate appropriately for pain, restlessness, or anxiety as prescribed and assess effect in 10 to 20 min.
3. Notify physician if:
   Paradoxical pulse greater than 10 mm Hg
   Systolic BP 90 mm Hg or less
   Urinary output 30 ml or less/hr
   Elevated "a" wave on RA pressure tracing during ventricular diastole
   CVP (RAP) greater than 8 torr or 15 mm H_2O
   PASP greater than 30 torr
   PADP greater than 12 or less than 5 torr
   PCWP greater than 12 or less than 5 torr
   Cardiac output less than 4.0 L/min
   Cardiac index less than 2.5 $L/min/m^2$
   SVR greater than 1200 units
   Onset of rales, dyspnea, respiratory distress
   Onset of electrical alternans or life-threatening arrhythmias
   Pulse pressure becomes progressively smaller
   Serum potassium greater than 6 mEq/L or less than 2.5 mEq/L
4. Anticipate physician to prescribe:
   Rapid IV infusion of saline, volume expanders
   Unloading IV medications to decrease SVR
   Medications for pain, anxiety, emesis

Pericardiocentesis to relieve intrapericardial pressure, and prevent
  cardiogenic shock
Intrapericardial injection of fluorouracil or thiophoramide
Histologic studies on aspirated pericardial fluid (do not discard!)
Insertion of temporary indwelling pericardial catheter
Surgical intervention for permanent pericardial pleural window to
  prevent future occurrence of pericardial effusion and tamponade
Radiation to control malignant pericardial effusion
Chemotherapy

BIBLIOGRAPHY

Adenle, A.D., and Edwards, J.E. Clinical and pathologic features of metastatic
  neoplasms of the pericardium. *Chest*, **81**(2), 1982, 166–169.
Boldt, M.A. *Acute coronary care*. New York: John Wiley and Sons, 1983.
Brantigan, C.O. Hemodynamic monitoring: Interpreting values. *American Journal
  of Nursing*, **82**(1), 1982, 86–89.
Corbett, J.V. *Laboratory tests in nursing practice*. Norwalk, Connecticut: Appleton-
  Century-Crofts, 1982.
Dracup, K.A., Breu, C.S., and Tillisch, J.H. Physiologic basis for combined
  nitroprusside—Dopamine therapy in postmyocardial infarction heart failure.
  Heart and Lung, **10**(1), 1981, 114–116.
Fletcher, B. *Quick reference to critical care nursing*. Philadelphia: J.B. Lippincott,
  1983, pp. 74–76.
Forrester, J.S., and Staniloff, H.M. Pericardial tamponade. *Emergency Medicine*,
  14(6), 1982, 64–75.
Gordon, M. *Manual of nursing diagnosis*. New York: McGraw-Hill, 1982.
Hudak, C.M., Lohr, T., and Gallo, B. *Critical care nursing*. Philadelphia: J.B.
  Lippincott, 1982.
Johanson, B.C., et al. *Standards for critical care*. St. Louis: C.V. Mosby, 1981.
Keck, S., et al. Cardiac tamponade. *Heart and Lung*, **12**(5), 1983, 505–509.
Kinnebrew, M.N. Add paradoxical pulse to your assessment routine. *RN*, **44**(11),
  1981, 32–33.
Kinney, M.R., et al. *A.A.C.N.'s clinical reference for critical care nursing*. New York:
  McGraw-Hill, 1981.
Luckman, J., and Sorensen, K.C. *Medical-surgical nursing—A psychophysiologic
  approach* (2nd ed.). Philadelphia: W.B. Saunders, 1980.
Marriott, H.J.L. *Practical electrocardiography* (6th ed.). Baltimore: Williams and
  Wilkins, 1977.
Norris, D.L., and Klein, L.A. What all those pressure readings mean . . . and why. *RN*,
  44(10), 1981, 35–41.
Pursley, P. Acute cardiac tamponade. *AJN*, **83**(10), 1983, 1414–1418.
Reynolds, S.F. Cardiac trauma and tamponade. *Critical Care Quarterly*, **23**(4), 1981,
  27–35.

Sweetwood, H. Cardiac tamponade—When dyspnea spells sudden death. *RN*, **43**(10), 1980, 35-41.

Theologides, A. Neoplastic cardiac tamponade. In J. Yarbro and R. Bornstein (Eds.), *Oncologic emergencies*. New York: Grune and Stratton 1981, pp. 1-21.

Wegman, J.A., and Forshee, T. Malignant pleural effusion: Pertinent issues. *Heart and Lung*, **12**(5), 1983, 533-543.

Yasko, J.M., and Schafer, S.L. Neoplastic pericardial tamponade. In *Guidelines for cancer care—Symptom management*. J.M. Yasko (Ed.), Virginia: Reston, 1983, pp. 343-346.

15. Constrictive Pericarditis

DEFINITION AND CAUSATIVE FACTORS

Pericarditis develops from an inflammation and scarring of the pericardium as a result of radiation therapy to the chest or invasion of the pericardial space by malignant tumors. Acute pericarditis is usually hallmarked by sharp chest pain referred to the back and shoulders and an elevation in the client's WBC count and temperature. Chronic constrictive pericarditis is manifested by systemic venous hypertension with right ventricular involvement and pulmonary congestion with left ventricular involvement. Pericardial inflammation causes the deposition of fibrin, producing restrictive adhesions that limit the filling capacity of the heart and consequently cardiac output. Inflammation can also result in the production of fluid in the pericardial space causing pericardial effusion (Chapter 14). The basic problem with pericarditis is ventricular filling rather than ventricular emptying. Pericarditis is characterized by elevated right atrial pressure and an early diastolic knock representing maximal ventricular filling early in diastole instead of throughout diastole which normally occurs.

Corresponding cancers include mesotheliomas, angiosarcomas, and metastatic tumors of the lung, breast, leukemias, Hodgkin, non-Hodgkin lymphoma, melanoma, ovaries, and GI primaries. Viral, fungal, and bacterial infections, chest trauma, acute myocardial infarctions, and uremia are additional causes.

ASSESSMENT DATA

- Pericardial friction rub—in systole and diastole
- Precordial chest pain—sharp, moderate to severe, referred to back and shoulders
- Tachycardia or atrial fibrillation
- Pulsus paradoxus in 50%
- Elevated WBC greater than 11,500/mm^3
- Fever, chills

- Absent PMI or difficult to locate
- Diastolic knock
- EKG—low voltage but normal QRS, ST elevation, or inverted T waves
- Right-sided failure
  Elevated CVP
  Equal right and left ventricular diastolic pressures
  Hepatomegaly
  Distended neck veins
  Edema, ascites
- Left-sided failure
  Rales, rhonchi, wheeze
  Gallop
  Dyspnea
  Hypotension
  Tachypnea
  Change in LOC
- Chest x-ray—heart is misshapened and calcifications are present

NURSING DIAGNOSES

Alteration in cardiac output, decreased, related to reduced ventricular end diastolic volume, decreased systolic blood pressure, and increased venous return.

RATIONALE

Cardiac output is decreased due to compression of the heart restricting the pumping action.

NURSING INTERVENTIONS

Monitoring–Independent

1. BP, heart rate, and respirations every 1 to 2 hr. Observe for narrowing pulse pressure.
2. Assess for pulsus paradoxus during each blood pressure measurement.
3. Auscultate heart sounds every 4 to 8 hr and record presence of friction rub—location and number of components.
4. Assess neck veins for distention in cm with HOB at 60° every 2 to 4 hr.
5. Auscultate all lung fields every 4 to 8 hr and record location and type of adventitious breath sounds.
6. Assess for SOB, dyspnea, orthopnea, and use of accessory muscles every 4 to 8 hr.

7. Assess client for pain with each contact and record location, intensity, radiation, onset during inspiration. Assess associated symptoms with each pain episode—nausea, vomiting, diaphoresis, anxiety, and skin color.

8. Assess cardiac rhythm and/or EKG for ST elevation (concave curvature) in leads I, II, III and V_{1-6}, flattened or inverted T wave in all leads but AVR. (ST elevation occurs first followed by return to baseline and T wave changes for acute pericarditis. When chronic, expect to see low voltage, flat, or inverted T waves, or atrial fibrillation.)

9. Oral temperature every 4 hr. Document if chills present or absent.

10. Palpate peripheral pulses for bilateral quality every 8 hr.

11. Assess for dependent edema every 8 hr.

12. Assess LOC q 8 hr and record changes in orientation, awareness, and behavior.

13. Assess skin color, temperature, and moisture every 4 to 8 hr.

14. Hourly urinary outputs, calculate I/O ratio for fluid balance every 8 and 24 hr.

15. Assess IV site for pain, redness, swelling q 4 to 8 hr.

Monitoring–Interdependent

1. Assess CVP measurements q 2 hr or as prescribed (if applicable) and compare to previous and normal values: 4 to 8 mm H_2O.
   (Other hemodynamic pressures may be apppropriate depending on severity of symptoms and condition.)

2. Assess laboratory data when available and compare to previous and normal values.
   ABGs pH: 7.35 to 7.45
           Po_2: 75 to 100 torr
           Pco_2: 35 to 45 torr
           HCO_3: 24 to 30 mEq/L
           O_2 Saturation: 95 to 100%
           BE: ± 2 mEq/L
           CO_2 Content: 24 to 30 mEq/L
   Serum Sodium: 135 to 145 mEq/L
   Serum Potassium: 3.5 to 5.0 mEq/L
   Serum Chloride: 100 to 106 mEq/L
   Serum Calcium: 8.5 to 10.5 mg/dl
   CBC Hemoglobin: 13.0 to 18.0 g/dl males
                        12.0 to 16.0 g/dl females
         Hematocrit: 45 to 52% males
                  37 to 48% females

RBC: 4.6 to 6.2 × 10⁶/mm³ males
      4.2 to 5.4 × 10⁶/mm³ females
MCH: 27 to 32 pg
MCHC: 32 to 36%
MCV: 80 to 94 cu microns
Platelets: 130,000 to 370,000 mm³
Prothrombin Time: control + 4 sec
Partial Thromboplastin Time: control + 10 sec
Lee-White Clotting Time: 6 to 17 min
WBC: 4,500 to 11,500/mm³

3. Assess effect of antiinflammatory medication using criteria of absence of pain and friction rub.

Change-Independent

1. HOB at 60° or position of maximum comfort.
2. Maintain bedrest and minimize physical exertion.
3. Humidified O_2 at 2 L/min or as prescribed.
4. Turn, cough, deep breathe q 2 hr.
5. Mouth care using soft toothbrush and mouthwash q 8 hr. Once a day, clean teeth with a mixture of H_2O_2 and baking soda to neutralize oral acid and remove plaque.
6. Passive ROME to all major joints q 4 hr while on bedrest.
7. Back care and massage all bony prominences with lotion q 4 hr.
8. Before all procedures, explain purpose and technique using understandable terms.
9. Reorient to time, place, reason for hospitalization if client confused or disoriented.
10. Eliminate all environmental safety hazards. Keep side rails up and pad if client restless or disoriented, place call light and personal articles within easy reach.
11. Explain condition and progress to client and family with each contact. Assist them to ask questions and express concerns of the present and the future.
12. Include family members in plan of care and allow them to participate, if mutually beneficial.

Change-Interdependent

1. D5W at KVO or as prescribed by physician.
2. Medicate appropriately for pain, as prescribed, and assess effect in 15 to 20 min.

3. Notify physician if:
    WBC greater than 10,000/mm³
    Oral temperature greater than 101.0° F
    Systolic blood pressure less than 90 torr
    Onset of ST and T wave changes consistent with pericarditis
    Onset of friction rub
4. Anticipate physician to prescribe:
    Steroids to minimize acute inflammation
    Diuretics to decrease circulatory volume and venous return
    Pericardiocentesis to relieve intrapericardial pressure with effusion
    Surgical release of pericardial constriction

BIBLIOGRAPHY

Corbett, J.V. *Laboratory tests in nursing practice.* Norwalk, Connecticut: Appleton-Century-Crofts, 1982.

Friedman, A.H. The diagnosis and management of life-threatening cardiac complications of cancer. In A.D. Turnbull (Ed.), *Current problems in cancer* (Vol. 4, No. 3). Chicago: Year Book Medical, 1979, pp. 30–33.

Gordon, M. *Manual of nursing diagnosis.* New York: McGraw-Hill, 1982.

Harvey, A.M., Johns, R.J., McKusick, V.A., Owens, A.H., and Ross, R.S. *The principles and practice of medicine* (20th ed.). New York: Appleton-Century-Crofts, 1980.

Horton, J., and Hill, G.J. *Clinical oncology.* Philadelphia: W.B. Saunders, 1977.

Johanson, B.C., et al. *Standards for critical care.* St. Louis: C.V. Mosby, 1981.

Luckman, J., and Sorensen, K.C. *Medical–surgical nursing—A psychophysiologic approach* (2nd ed.). Philadelphia: W.B. Saunders, 1980.

Marriott, H.J.L. *Practical electrocardiography* (6th ed.). Baltimore: Williams and Wilkins, 1977.

16. Chemotherapy Related Cardiomyopathy

DEFINITION AND CAUSATIVE FACTORS

Chemotherapy-induced cardiomyopathy is characterized by a pale, flabby myocardium with ventricular dilatation and hypertrophy, and not uncommonly biatrial enlargement. Fibrosis, pericardial effusion, and mural, pulmonary, and systemic thrombi are frequent coexisting conditions. Congestive heart failure is evidence of the cardiomyopathic process, but critical degeneration of the myocardium precedes any indication of heart failure. There is a reduction in the number of myocardial fibrils which limits the contractile function. As a result, left ventricular end diastolic pressure (LVEDP) increases and ejection fraction and stroke volume (cardiac output) decreases. The workload of the heart is great because the increased intraventricular tension resulting from the dilated chamber causes an increased demand for oxygen. Cardiac output can be maintained for a time with compensatory tachycardia, but there is no cardiac reserve for activity or stress. Congestive heart failure with right-sided involvement occurs as pulmonary hypertension develops with an increasing LVEDP.

Coronary arteries and heart valves are usually not involved. Corresponding cancers include all those treated with chemotherapy and mediastinal radiation. The following chemotherapeutic agents are cardiotoxic producing arrhythmias and cardiomyopathy with long-term use.

Adriamycin: dose of greater than or equal to 200 mg/m^2 with increasing frequency in doses greater than or equal to 550 mg/m^2

Cytoxan: synergistic effect with Adriamycin

Doxorubicin with adjuvant radiation therapy to the mediastinum

Cumulative effect with any of the above drugs and either vincristine, actinomycin D, or mithramycin

ASSESSMENT DATA

- Cardiac arrhythmias
  Atrial fibrillation
  Supraventricular tachycardias
  Ventricular and atrial ectopy
- EKG changes
  Left axis deviation
  Nonspecific T wave changes
  Bundle branch block
  Large notched P waves
- CHF
  Rales, rhonchi, wheeze
  Tachycardia
  Orthopnea
  Tachypnea
  Pulmonary edema
  Gallop rhythm
  Decreased LOC
  Fatigue
- Right-sided failure
  Distended neck veins
  Hepatomegaly
  Peripheral edema
- Hemodynamic changes
  Increased right atrial pressure (CVP)
  Increased pulmonary artery pressure (PAP)
  Increased pulmonary capillary wedge pressure (PCWP)
  Decreased cardiac output/index
  Decreased blood pressure
- X-ray—enlarged heart

NURSING DIAGNOSES

Alteration in cardiac output, decreased, related to an enlarged heart with ineffective pumping action, resulting in an increased LVEDP, decreased cardiac output and pulmonary hypertension.

RATIONALE

Certain chemotherapeutic drugs cause cardiac dilatation with ventricular hypertrophy. This limits the contractile function of the heart, thus decreasing cardiac output

NURSING INTERVENTIONS

Monitoring–Independent

1. BP, heart rate, and respirations q 1 to 2 hr, q 15 to 30 min if condition life-threatening.
2. Assess heart sounds in all 4 valvular sites and record location of PMI and gallop q 4 to 8 hr.
3. Assess neck vein distention in cm with HOB at 60° q 4 to 8 hr.
4. Assess cardiac monitor for
   Cardiac arrhythmias
   T wave changes
   Bundle branch block
   P wave notching
   Document time and change with a rhythm strip
5. Assess LOC q 4 to 8 hr and record changes in awareness, orientation, and behavior.
6. Palpate peripheral pulses for bilateral quality q 8 hr.
7. Assess for peripheral edema q 8 hr.
8. Assess skin color, temperature, and moisture with each client contact.
9. Hourly urine output and calculate I/0 ratio for fluid balance q 8 and 24 hr.
10. Auscultate lung sounds in all fields, symmetry of chest expansion, and use of accessory muscles, q 4 to 8 hr, and record onset of rales, wheeze, and rhonchi.
11. Assess for dyspnea, orthopnea, tachypnea with each client contact.
12. Temperature q 4 hr.
13. Assess IV site for redness, swelling, and pain q 4 to 8 hr.

Monitoring–Interdependent

1. Assess hemodynamic pressure measurements after insertion of pulmonary artery flotation catheter (Swan–Ganz) and compare to previous and normal values (frequency depends on agency protocol or as prescribed by physician).

	NORMAL	CARDIOMYOPATHY
PASP	20–30 torr	Increases
PADP	7–12 torr	Increases
PCWP	8–12 torr	Increases
Cardiac output	4–8 L/min	Decreases
Cardiac index	3.5 ± 0.7 L/min/m²	Decreases
CVP	0–5 torr	Increases

2. Assess laboratory data when available and compare to previous and normal values.

  ABGs   pH: 7.35 to 7.45

            Po_2: 75 to 100 torr

            Pco_2: 35 to 45 torr

            HCO_3: 24 to 30 mEq/L

            O_2 Saturation: 95 to 100%

            BE: ± 2 mEq/L

            CO_2 Content: 24 to 30 mEq/L

  Serum Sodium: 135 to 145 mEq/L

  Serum Potassium: 3.5 to 5.0 mEq/L

  Serum Chloride: 100 to 106 mEq/L

  Serum Calcium: 8.5 to 10.5 mg/dl

  BUN: 8 to 25 mg/dl

  Creatinine: 0.6 to 1.5 mg/dl

  CBC   Hemoglobin: 13.0 to 18.0 g/dl males

                      12.0 to 16.0 g/dl females

           Hematocrit: 45 to 52% males

                     37 to 48% females

           RBC: 4.6 to 6.2 × 10^6/mm^3 males

                   4.2 to 5.4 × 10^6/mm^3 females

  MCH: 27 to 32 pg

  MCHC: 32 to 36%

  MCV: 80 to 94 cu microns

  Platelets: 130,000 to 370,000 mm^3

  WBC: 4,500 to 11,500/mm^3

3. Assess effects of unloading medications if prescribed.

  Nipride to decrease preload and afterload by vasodilatation

  Dopamine to increase velocity and force of contraction, ejection fraction, stroke volume, renal vasodilatation, and to decrease SVR (afterload)

  Lasix to diurese excess fluid volume, reduce afterload, venous return, and pulmonary hypertension

Digoxin to increase force of contraction and improve cardiac output

Change–Independent

1. Humidified O_2 at 2 L/min by nasal cannula or as prescribed.
2. HOB at 45 to 60° or position of greatest comfort.
3. Maintain on bedrest and minimize all physical activity.
4. Turn, cough, deep breathe if tolerance permits q 2 to 4 hr.
5. Passive ROME to all major joints q 4 hr if tolerated.

6. Back care with friction massage to all bony prominences q 2 to 4 hr.

7. Mouth care using soft toothbrush and mouthwash or other oral antiseptic q 4 to 8 hr. Once a day, clean teeth with a mixture of H_2O_2 and baking soda to neutralize oral acid and remove plaque.

8. Eliminate all environmental hazards to safety. Keep side rails up and pad if client restless or disoriented. Place call light and personal articles within easy reach.

9. Before all procedures, explain purpose and technique in understandable terms.

10. Reorient to time, place, and reason for hospitalization if client confused or disoriented.

11. Maintain frequent visual and physical contact with client during life-threatening episodes stating time of return before leaving.

12. Explain condition and progress to client and family with each contact. Assist them to ask questions and express concerns of the present and the future.

13. Include family members in plan of care and allow them to participate, if mutually beneficial, once critical stage resolved.

Change–Interdependent

1. D5W at KVO or as prescribed by physician.

2. Medicate appropriately for pain, anxiety, or restlessness as prescribed and assess effect in 10 to 20 min.

3. Notify physician if:
    Systolic blood pressure less than 90 torr
    Urinary output less than 30 ml/hr
    PASP greater than 30 torr
    PADP greater than 12 torr
    PCWP greater than 18 torr
    CVP greater than 8 torr or 15 mm H_2O
    Cardiac output less than 4.0 L/min
    Cardiac index less than 2.5 L/min/m^2
    Onset of rales, dyspnea, or respiratory distress
    Onset of life-threatening arrhythmias
    Po_2 less than 75 torr
    Serum potassium greater than 6 mEq/L or less than 2.5 mEq/L

4. Anticipate physician to prescribe:
    Unloading medications to decrease preload
    Vasodilators to decrease afterload
    Cardiotonic medications to increase force of contraction
    Diuretics to decrease venous return and pulmonary hypertension

Heparin to prevent thromboemboli

Pericardiocentesis if pericardial effusion occurs due to greatly enlarged heart

Dialysis with kidney failure due to decreased renal perfusion from inadequate cardiac output

Discontinuation, reduction, or change in chemotherapy protocol

Discontinuation, reduction, or change in radiotherapy administration

---

BIBLIOGRAPHY

Breu, C.S., Lindenmuth, J.E., and Tillisch, J.H. Treatment of patients with congestive cardiomyopathy during hospitalization. A case study. *Heart and Lung*, 11(3), 1982, 229–235.

Corbett, J.V. *Laboratory tests in nursing practice*. Norwalk, Connecticut: Appleton-Century-Crofts, 1982.

Dracup, K.A., Breu, C.S., and Tillisch, J.H. Physiologic basis for combined nitroprusside–dopamine therapy in postmyocardial infarction heart failure. *Heart and Lung*, 10(1), 1981, 114–116.

Friedman, M.A., and Carter, S.K. Serious toxicities associated with chemotherapy. In J. Yarbro and R. Bornstein (Eds.), *Oncologic emergencies*. New York: Grune and Stratton, 1981, 119–139.

Gordon, M. *Manual of nursing diagnosis*. New York: McGraw-Hill, 1982.

Gottdiener, J.S., et al. Late effects of therapeutic mediastinal irradiation: Assessment by echocardiography and radionuclide angiography. *New England Journal of Medicine*, 308, 1983, 569–572.

Marriott, H.J.L. *Practical electrocardiography* (6th ed.). Baltimore: Williams and Wilkins, 1977.

Norris, D.L., and Klein, L.A. What all those pressure readings mean . . . and why. *RN*, 44(10), 1981, 35–41.

Wold, B. Dilated (congestive) cardiomyopathy: Considerations for the coronary care unit nurse. *Heart and Lung*, 12(5), 1983, 544–551.

17. Thrombophlebitis

DEFINITION AND CAUSATIVE FACTORS

Thrombophlebitis is an inflammation of a vein with clot formation caused by venous stasis, hypercoagulability, or injury to the venous endothelium. Clients with cancer have a greater potential for developing thrombophlebitis because of thromboplastin-like substances believed to be released from cancer cells, increased platelet and fibrinogen turnover rates, and elevated levels of factor V and VIII that participate in the clotting process. Intravenous chemotherapy is also a contributing factor. The normal coagulation process consists of the following events:

1. Vascular injury → release of tissue thromboplastin
2. Thromboplastin + 7 factors + prothrombin → thrombin
3. Thrombin + fibrinogen → fibrin
4. Fibrin + platelets → clot formation
5. Fibrinolysin → clot degradation

Thrombophlebitis is the most common manifestation of hypercoagulability disorders seen in the client with cancer, and DIC, cerebral venous thrombosis, and pulmonary thromboemboli are the most serious sequelae. Some authors (Ackerman and del Regato, 1970; Abeloff, 1979) report that thrombophlebitis is one of the first indications of malignancy, and once the primary tumor has been removed successfully, thrombophlebitic episodes disappear completely. Because of the higher risk of thrombophlebitis in patients with cancer, especially those who have had surgery, assessment of vein involvement should be standard nursing practice. The veins most commonly involved are the deep veins in the legs and those in the pelvis. Thrombophlebitis of arm veins can occur but the danger of emboli is rare.

Corresponding cancers include: bowel, pancreas, lung, prostate, stomach, lymphoma, leukemia, breast, and ovary. Advanced age, decreased mobility, heart disease, obesity, and abdominal pelvic surgery are additional causes.

ASSESSMENT DATA

- Positive Homan sign
- Pain, redness, swelling of calf or leg
- Abdominal pain on deep palpation
- Increased clotting time, partial thromboplastin time, thrombin time, fibrinogen, and prothrombin time
- Decreased, unequal, or absent peripheral pulses
- Neck vein distention
- Peripheral edema
- Prolonged immobilization
- Recent surgery
- IV chemotherapy
- Sudden onset of chest pain, dyspnea, cough, hemoptysis
- Sudden onset of headache, motor, sensory, speech deficits, visual disturbances, seizures, and altered LOC

NURSING DIAGNOSES	RATIONALE
Alterations in tissue perfusion, decreased, related to obstruction of venous return, emboli formation, and arterial insufficiency.	*Increase in fibrinogen, factors V and VIII, and thromboplastin lead to hypercoagulability. Surgery and IV chemotherapy are additional factors that may roughen the vein lining allowing platelets to adhere to it.*

Associated Nursing Diagnoses

1. Potential impaired gas exchange, related to pulmonary venous obstruction of alveoli, dysfunction, and collapse of alveoli.	Pulmonary thromboemboli is a sequela of hypercoagulability. Valvular insufficiency and muscular insufficiency decrease blood flow impairing gas exchange.
2. Potential sensory deficit—vision, motor, touch, related to obstruction of cerebral venous return, causing neurologic deficits.	Thromboembolic infarction of the central nervous system and/or migration of thrombi to the brain due to increased venous pressure or anticlotting factors in the blood.

NURSING INTERVENTIONS

Monitoring–Independent

1. Assess both leg calves for redness, tenderness q 8 hr.
2. Measure each leg calf and ankle at the fullest thickness or according to predetermined reference points q 8 hr.
3. Assess all peripheral pulses for bilateral equality—temporal, radial, brachial, femoral, popliteal, dorsalis pedal, and posterior tibial.
4. Assess for Homan sign in both legs q 8 hr except if signs of thrombophlebitis exist (Homan maneuver can dislodge a thrombus to become an embolus).
5. Assess IV site for redness, pain, and swelling q 4 to 8 hr.
6. Auscultate breath sounds in all lung fields, symmetry of chest expansion, and use of accessory muscles q 8 hr and record onset of adventitious sounds.
7. Document sudden onset of chest, abdominal, or pelvic pain and assess location, intensity, and aggravating and alleviating factors.
8. Inspect all sputum for hemoptysis.
9. Assess for dyspnea, SOB, tachypnea, hyperpnea q 2 hr with onset of thrombophlebitis, q 8 hr without overt signs.
10. Assess neck vein distention in cm with HOB at 45° q 8 hr.
11. Oral temperature q 4 hr.
12. Assess skin color, temperature, and moisture q 8 hr.
13. Blood pressure, heart rate q 2 hr with onset of thrombophlebitis, q 4 hrs otherwise.
14. Assess neurologic status q 4 to 8 hr and include
    LOC
    Behavior
    Motor coordination and strength
    Visual disturbances
    Speech and verbal articulation
    Seizure activity
    Headache
15. Accurate I and O and calculate I/O ratio for fluid balance q 8 and 24 hr.
16. Assess position of client. Fowler position is NOT recommended as it increases pooling of blood to pelvis and lower extremities.

Monitoring–Interdependent

1. Assess laboratory data when available and compare to normal values.
    Prothrombin Time: control + 4 sec
    Partial Thromboplastin Time: control + 10 sec

Fibrinogen: 200 to 500 mg/dl
Lee–White Clotting Time: 6 to 17 min
MCH: 27 to 32 pg
MCHC: 32 to 36%
MCV: 80 to 94 cu micron
RBC: 4.6 to 6.2 × 10^6/mm^3 males
    4.2 to 5.4 × 10^6/mm^3 females

2. Note results of chest x-ray, lung scan, pulmonary angiogram, when available.
3. Assess for signs of bleeding with heparin therapy.
    Hemocult all stools, emesis, urine q 8 hr
    Bruising
    Epistaxis
    Oral cavity bleeding
    Oozing from venipunctures
    Hemoglobin: 13 to 18 g/dl males
                12 to 16 g/dl females
    Hematocrit: 45 to 52% males
             37 to 48% females
    Platelets: 130,000 to 370,000 mm^3

Change–Independent

1. ROME to all unaffected major joints q 4 hr.
2. Bedrest and elevate limb on one pillow or elevate foot of bed 30°.
3. Apply footboard and teach footboard exercises for unaffected limb q 2 to 4 hr.
4. Force fluids to 150 ml q 1 hr while awake.
5. With anticoagulant therapy
    Apply direct pressure to all venipuncture sites × 10 min or until bleeding stops. Place sandbag over bone marrow aspiration site.
    Coordinate laboratory work to minimize unnecessary venipunctures.
    File fingernails to shortest length and soft brush clean qd
6. Turn, cough, deep breathe q 2 hr while on bedrest.
7. Lightly massage to all bony prominences q 4 hr.
8. Mouth care using soft toothbrush and mouthwash pc. Once a day, clean teeth with a mixture of H_2O_2 and baking soda to neutralize oral acid and remove plaque
9. Eliminate all environmental hazards to safety. Keep side rails up and pad if client restless or disoriented, place bed in low position, and place call light and personal articles within easy reach.

10. Before all procedures, explain purpose and technique in understandable terms.
11. Reorient to time, place, and reason for hospitalization if client disoriented or confused.
12. Assist client to perform ADLs and maintain judicious independence and control over self and environment within physical limitations.
13. Explain condition and progress to client and family with each contact. Assist them to ask questions and express concerns of the present and the future.
14. Include family members in plan of care and allow them to participate, if mutually therapeutic.
15. Teach client receiving anticoagulant therapy to
    Eliminate nose trauma by blowing, picking
    Eliminate straining during defecation
    Use electric razor for shaving
    Eliminate toothpicks, dental floss, and tampon use

Change–Interdependent

1. D5W at KVO or heparin lock or as prescribed by physician.
2. Medicate appropriately for pain and assess effect in 10 to 20 min.
3. Notify physician if:
    Client experiences leg pain with redness and swelling
    Client develops sudden onset of chest pain with temperature elevation, dyspnea, cough
    Sudden onset of headache and other neurologic deficits, or deep pelvic pain
    IV site has redness, pain, or swelling
    With heparin therapy
       Hematocrit less than 35%
       Hemoglobin less than 10 g/dl
       BP systolic less than 90 torr
       Active, profuse bleeding occurs from any site
4. Anticipate the physician to prescribe:
    Heparin: to decrease thrombin activity and prevent new clots or extension of clots from occurring
    Aspirin: to decrease "stickiness" of cancer cells
    Persantine: to decrease cell "stickiness"
    Hot packs to affected leg
    Antacids to prevent gastric irritation from aspirin
    Stool softeners to prevent bowel irritation from impaction of stool
    TED hose prophylactically to unaffected leg

6 to 8 inch shock blocks to foot of bed to increase venous return and
prevent venous stasis
Alternate site and/or route for administration of chemotherapy

BIBLIOGRAPHY

Ackerman, L.V., and del Regato, J.A. *Cancer: Diagnosis, treatment, and prognosis.*
St. Louis: C.V. Mosby, 1970.
Abeloff, M.D. (Ed.). *Complications of cancer.* Baltimore: The Johns Hopkins Uni-
versity Press, 1979, pp. 121–145.
Brown, S. Venous thrombosis: Another complication of cancer. *Oncology Nursing
Forum,* 10(2), 1983, 41–47.
Burns, N. *Nursing and cancer.* Philadelphia: W.B. Saunders, 1982, pp. 241–242.
Caprini, J.A., and Sener, S.F. Altered coagulability in cancer patients. *CA-A Cancer
Journal for Clinicians,* (3), 1981, 162–172.
Crobett, J.V. *Laboratory Tests in Nursing Practice.* Norwalk, Connecticut: Appleton-
Century-Crofts, 1982.
Gordon, M. *Manual of Nursing Diagnosis.* New York: McGraw-Hill, 1982.
Hasegawa, D.K., and Bloomfield, C.D. Thrombotic and hemorrhagic manifestations
of malignancy. In J. Yarbro and R. Bornstein (Eds.), *Oncologic emergencies.* New
York: Grune and Stratton, 1981, pp. 165–167.
Hickey, W.F., Garnick, M.B., Henderson, I.C., and Dawson, D.M. Primary cerebral
venous thrombosis in patients with cancer—A rarely diagnosed paraneoplastic
syndrome. *The American Journal of Medicine,* 73, 1982, 740–750.
Taylor, D.L. Thrombophlebitis: Physiology, signs, and symptoms. *Nursing '83,* 13(7),
1983, 52–53.
Wajima, T. Thrombophlebitis in Cancer Patients. *Annals of the New York Academy
of Sciences,* 370, 1981, 138–144.

18. Airway Obstruction

DEFINITION AND CAUSATIVE FACTORS

Airway obstruction can occur in any segment of the respiratory tract as a result of an in situ tumor or metastasis from adjacent structures. The degree of obstruction depends on its location and the extent of lumen narrowing. Obstruction of the larynx and trachea are usually slow in developing and are preceded by preliminary warnings, notably shortness of breath. Primary tumors of the trachea (rare) and larynx (common) and secondary tumors of the neck and lungs are the causative factors for upper airway obstruction. Bronchogenic carcinomas, and less often metastasis from other sites, are responsible for lower airway obstruction, and dyspnea is most often the presenting symptom. The onset of lower respiratory tract obstruction is usually sudden because the bronchial or bronchiolar lumen is smaller, and even small endobronchial tumors can cause distal collapse of the bronchial tree resulting in impaired pulmonary function. Diagnosis is made by x-ray, bronchoscopy, and sputum cytology.

Corresponding cancers include tongue base, pharynx, larynx, thyroid, bronchus, lung, and esophagus. Mediastinal tumors, Waldeyer ring (pharynx) involvement associated with leukemia and lymphoma, chronic graft–versus–host disease (Chapter 27), COPD, pneumonia, and superior vena cava syndrome (Chapter 13) are additional causes.

ASSESSMENT DATA

- SOB
- Dyspnea*
- Wheezing, stridor, snoring, crowing breath sounds
- Orthopnea, tachypnea

---

*Dyspnea in clients with acute or chronic myeloblastic leukemia may be due to a reduction in their WBC count resulting from oral intake of hydroxyurea (50 mg/kg/day) or from centrifugation leukophoresis.

- Retraction and use of accessory muscles
- Bilateral vocal cord paralysis with neck in adducted position
- Tachycardia
- Unilateral neck vein distention
- Pale, cool, moist skin progressing to cyanosis
- X-ray, bronchoscopy, and sputum cytology indicating obstruction

NURSING DIAGNOSES	RATIONALE
Ineffective airway clearance, related to partial or complete respiratory tract obstruction, resulting from tumor invasion, extension, or primary carcinoma.	*Primary or secondary tumor invasion of the respiratory tract causes blockage of the airway which comprises adequate pulmonary and cardiac function.*

NURSING INTERVENTIONS

Monitoring–Independent

1. Auscultate breath sounds in all lung fields q 4 to 8 hr and record onset of diminished, absent, or adventitious sounds. With onset of SOB or dyspnea, assess q 1 to 2 hr.
2. Assess symmetry of chest expansion, depth, and rate of inspiration, and use of accessory muscles with each auscultation.
3. Assess client for SOB, dyspnea, and cough with each contact.
4. Inspect all sputum for hemoptysis.
5. Assess LOC q 8 hr and record changes in awareness, orientation, and behavior.
6. Assess skin color, temperature, and moisture q 4 to 8 hr.
7. Assess for neck vein distention in cm q 8 hr.
8. Rectal temperature q 4 hr.
9. Palpate peripheral pulses for bilateral quality q 8 hr.
10. Auscultate heart sounds in 4 valvular sites q 4 to 8 hr and record onset of gallop.
11. BP, heart rate, respirations q 2 hr.
12. Hourly I and O and calculate I/O ratio for fluid balance q 8 and 24 hr.
13. Assess IV site for redness, swelling, and pain q 4 to 8 hr.

Monitoring–Interdependent

1. Assess laboratory data when available and compare to previous and normal values.

   ABGs pH: 7.35 to 7.45

          Po_2: 75 to 100 torr

          Pco_2: 35 to 45 torr

          HCO_3: 24 to 30 mEq/L

          O_2 Saturation: 95 to 100%

          BE: ± 2 mEq/L

          CO_2 Content: 24 to 30 mEq/L

   CBC Hemoglobin: 13.0 to 18.0 g/dl males

                   12.0 to 16.0 g/dl females

          Hematocrit: 45 to 52% males

                   37 to 48% females

          RBC: 4.6 to $6.2 \times 10^6/mm^3$ males

              4.2 to $5.4 \times 10^6/mm^3$ females

          MCH: 27 to 32 pg

          MCHC: 32 to 36%

          MCV: 80 to 94 cu microns

          WBC: 4,500 to $11,500/mm^3$

          Platelets: 130,000 to 370,000 mm^3

2. Assess results of serial chest x-rays, bronchoscopy, and sputum cytology when available.

Change–Independent

1. Position HOB at 60 to 90°
2. Humidified O_2 at 2 L/min by nasal cannula or as prescribed by physician.
3. Maintain bedrest with minimized activity schedule.
4. Turn, cough, deep breathe q 2 hr.
5. Mouth care using an oral antiseptic q 4 hr, if client NPO. Once a day, clean teeth with a mixture of H_2O_2 and baking soda to neutralize oral acid and remove plaque.
6. Passive ROME to all major joints q 4 hr.
7. Back care and massage all bony prominences with lotion q 4 hr.
8. Eliminate all irritating inhalants from environment

       Strong cleaning solutions

       Tobacco smoke (visitors and client)

       Heavy scents in personal toiletries

       Aerosols

9. Isolate client from others (visitors, staff, clients) with any infectious process during acute phase.

10. Maintain frequent physical and visual contact during acute phase stating time of return before leaving.

11. Before all procedures, explain purpose and technique in understandable terms.

12. Eliminate all environmental safety hazards. Keep side rails up and pad if client confused or restless, place call light and personal articles within easy reach.

13. Explain condition and progress to client and family with each contact. Assist them to ask questions and express concerns of the present and the future.

14. Include family members in plan of care and allow them to participate, if mutually beneficial.

Change–Interdependent

1. D5W at KVO or as prescribed by physician.

2. Medicate appropriately for pain or anxiety and assess effect in 10 to 20 min.

3. Notify physician if:
   Dyspnea, SOB, or respiratory distress occurs
   pH less than 7.35
   Po_2 less than 75 torr
   Pco_2 greater than 45 torr (uncompensated)
   O_2 saturation less than 90%
   Hemoglobin less than 10 g/dl
   Hematocrit less than 30%
   WBC count less than $4,000/mm^3$ in clients with myeloblastic leukemia

4. Anticipate physician to prescribe:
   Bronchoscopy to diagnose location of obstruction
   Radiation to reduce size of tumor
   Chemotherapy
   Tracheostomy if obstruction proximal to trachea
   Broad spectrum antibiotics to minimize risk of secondary infection
   Bronchodilators to increase lumen size
   Surgical removal of obstructing tumor
   (Intubation is usually contraindicated.)

BIBLIOGRAPHY

Corbett, J.V. *Laboratory tests in nursing practice.* Norwalk, Connecticut: Appleton-Century-Crofts, 1982.

Gordon, M. *Manual of nursing diagnosis.* New York: McGraw-Hill, 1982.

Hall, J.P., and Jackson, V.D. Adult respiratory medical emergencies. *Nursing Clinics of North America,* **16**(1), 1981, 75–83.

Kinney, M.R., et al. *A.A.C.N.'s clinical reference for critical care nursing.* New York: McGraw-Hill, 1981.

Luckman, J., and Sorensen, K.C. *Medical-surgical nursing—A psychophysiologic approach* (2nd ed.). Philadelphia: W.B. Saunders, 1980.

Morrison, M.L. *Respiratory intensive care nursing* (2nd ed.). Boston: Little, Brown, 1979.

Roca, J. et al. Fatal airway disease in an adult with chronic graft–versus–host disease. *Thorax,* **37**, 1982, 77–78.

Sise, J.G., and Crichlow, R.W. Obstruction due to malignant tumors. In J. Yarbro and R. Bornstein (Eds.), *Oncologic emergencies.* New York: Grune and Stratton, 1981, pp. 97–118.

Strong, E.W. Head and neck emergencies—Airway obstruction. In A.D. Turnbull (Ed.), *Current problems in cancer* (Vol. 4, No. 3). Chicago: Year Book Medical Publishers, Inc., September 1979, pp. 36–39.

Witkowski, J.A., and Lawrence, C.P. Bazex's syndrome—Paraneoplastic acrokeratosis. *The Journal of the American Medical Association,* **248**(21), 1982, 2883–2884.

19. Aspiration Pneumonia

DEFINITION AND CAUSATIVE FACTORS

Aspiration pneumonitis (Mendelson syndrome) occurs as a result of vomiting or regurgitation of stomach contents. Regurgitation is a silent, passive process related to an increased gastric pressure gradient when the cough and epiglottis reflex are depressed. Vomiting is an active process, and the indications are usually evident. The more acidic the aspirant, the greater the damage. Degeneration of the bronchial epithelium and alveolar cells and increased alveolar epithelial permeability causes exudation of intravascular fluid, RBCs, and protein, producing edematous, hemorrhagic alveoli. Atelectasis, hypoxia, and acidosis are the end results. Aspiration pneumonia is a primary cause of adult respiratory distress syndrome (ARDS), with a characteristic latent period between the occurrence of aspiration and onset of hypoxic symptoms. ARDS (wet lung, shock lung, white lung, adult hyaline membrane disease) is characterized by a reduction in functional residual capacity and lung volume and decreasing pulmonary compliance due to interstitial and interalveolar edema, microemboli, atelectasis, and thickened and necrosed alveolar walls.

Corresponding cancers include all those being treated with chemotherapy (but there is a greater risk with vincristine), esophageal, larynx cancers, and multiple myeloma (due to decreased antibody response). Excessive sedation, clogged NG tubes, tracheostomy and endotracheal tubes, debilitated, uremic, or comatose clients, and severe vomiting are additional causes.

ASSESSMENT DATA

- Uncharacteristic tracheal suctioned secretions
- Hyperpnea, tachypnea, dyspnea
- Intercostal and supracostal retractions
- Stridor
- Restlessness, anxiety, and change in LOC

- Rales, rhonchi, wheeze, cough
- Decreased or absent breath sounds
- Dullness on chest percussion
- Fever
- Chest pain—stabbing or increased by coughing
- Chest x-ray—lungs look white (late sign)
- ABGs   Increased Pco_2
          Decreased Po_2
          Decreased pH
- WBC—elevated with infection

NURSING DIAGNOSES

Impaired gas exchange, related to a decrease in functioning alveoli and decreased functional residual capacity, lung volume, and pulmonary compliance.

RATIONALE

Increased permeability of alveolar epithelium to aspirated contents of stomach causes pulmonary compromise.

NURSING INTERVENTIONS

Monitoring–Independent

1. Auscultate breath sounds in all lung fields q 8 hr and record onset of diminished, absent, adventitious sounds, or friction rub q 1 hr if aspiration suspected or with onset of symptoms.
2. Percuss all lung fields q 4 hr and record onset of dullness.
3. Assess for hyperpnea, tachypnea, and dyspnea with each contact.
4. Assess use of accessory muscles and symmetry of chest expansion q 4 hr.
5. Inspect all sputum for hemoptysis, specifically pink, frothy sputum.
6. Assess for nausea and vomiting with each client contact.
7. Assess LOC q 8 hr and record changes in awareness, orientation, and behavior.
8. Assess skin temperature, color, and moisture q 2 to 4 hr.
9. Rectal temperature q 4 hr, q 2 hr with elevation.
10. Auscultate heart sounds in 4 valvular sites q 8 hr and record onset of gallop or murmur.
11. Assess for neck vein distention in cm with HOB at 60° q 8 hr.

12. Palpate peripheral pulses for bilateral quality q 8 hr.
13. Hourly I and O and calculate I/O ratio for fluid balance q 8 and 24 hr.
14. Blood pressure, heart rate, and respirations q 2 hr.
15. Assess bowel sounds in all 4 quadrants q 4 to 8 hr and record onset of abdominal distention and rebound tenderness.
16. Assess IV site for redness, pain, swelling q 4 to 8 hr.

Monitoring–Interdependent

1. Assess laboratory data when available and compare to previous and normal values.
   ABGs   pH: 7.35 to 7.45
               Po_2: 75 to 100 torr
               Pco_2: 35 to 45 torr
               HCO_3: 24 to 30 mEq/L
               CO_2 Content: 24 to 30 mEq/L
               O_2 Saturation: 95 to 100%
   WBC: 4,500 to 11,500/mm^3
   Serum potassium: 3.5 to 5.0 mEq/L
2. Note results of chest x-ray when available.
3. Assess patency of N/G tube if applicable.
4. Measure pH of gastric secretions via N/G tube q 8 hr.
5. Assess ventilator settings for prescribed:
   Tidal volume 12 to 15 ml/kg recommended
   Inspiratory pressure
   Rate—compare number of spontaneous respirations to mechanical ventilations with IMV (intermittent mandatory ventilation)
   FIO_2 percent
   PEEP in cm. If CPPV (continuous positive pressure volume) is used with PEEP, assess for pneumothorax q 4 hr; tracheal shift, asymmetrical chest expansion, respiratory distress, and absence of breath sounds.
6. Measure MOV (minimal occlusive volume) of tracheal cuff q 8 hr and record.
7. Assess residual of intermittent tube feedings before administering and omit if greater than 100 ml. Assess stomach for emptying ability with continuous tube feeding q 4 hr.

Change–Independent

1. Elevate HOB to 45 to 90° if client is NOT semicomatosed or comatosed.
2. Humidified O_2 at 2 L/min by nasal cannula or oxygen delivery, as determined by physician.
3. Maintain bedrest and minimize activity with onset of respiratory distress.

4. Turn, cough, deep breathe q 2 hr.

5. Passive ROME q 4 hr while on bedrest.

6. Back care and massage to all bony prominences with lotion q 4 hr.

7. Mouth care using an oral antiseptic q 4 hr if client NPO. Once a day, clean teeth with a mixture of H_2O_2 and baking soda to neutralize oral acid and remove plaque.

8. Force fluids to 150 ml q 1 hr alternating between water and juice if po fluids appropriate.

9. Gradual activity schedule q 4 hr or as prescribed by physician.

10. Maintain frequent physical and visual contact with client during acute onset of symptoms and q hr if ventilator used, stating time of return before leaving.

11. Reorient to time, place, and reason for hospitalization with each contact if client confused or disoriented.

12. Before all procedures, explain purpose and technique using understandable terms.

13. Eliminate all environmental safety hazards. Keep side rails up and pad if client restless or confused, place call light and personal articles within easy reach.

14. Assist client to perform ADLs and maintain judicious independence over self and environment within physical limitations.

15. Explain condition and progress to client and family with each contact. Assist them to ask questions and express concerns of the present and the future.

16. Include family members in plan of care and allow them to participate if mutually therapeutic.

Change–Interdependent

1. D5W at KVO or as prescribed.

2. Medicate appropriately for pain or anxiety and assess effects in 10 to 20 min.

3. Notify physician if:
   ABGs within normal range but respiratory distress evident (indicates inadequate ventilation)
   pH less than 7.35
   Po_2 less than 70 torr
   Pco_2 greater than 45 torr
   O_2 saturation less than 90%
   Serum potassium greater than 6 mEq/L
   Onset of severe rales, rhonchi, wheeze, or absence of breath sounds
   Rectal temperature greater than 101.0° F.

Increasing MOV

Evidence of inadequate stomach emptying with continuous or intermittent tube feedings

4. Anticipate the physician to prescribe:

Tagamet: to increase gastric fluid pH

Steroids and heparin, although considered controversial in therapeutic value

Broad spectrum antibiotics—alveoli distal to atelectasis in danger of infection

BIBLIOGRAPHY

Ciresi, S.A. Pulmonary aspiration: A review. *Journal of the American Association of Nurse Anesthetists,* **50**(6), 1982, 266–269.

Corbett, J.V. *Laboratory tests in nursing practice.* Norwalk, Connecticut: Appleton-Century-Crofts, 1982.

Gordon, M. *Manual of nursing diagnosis.* New York: McGraw-Hill, 1982.

Hardesty, G.A. Prevention of aspiration pneumonitis: Preoperative preparation. *Journal of the American Association of Nurse Anesthetists,* **49**(2), 1981, 52–54.

Kinney, M.R., et al. *A.A.C.N.'s clinical reference for critical care nursing.* New York: McGraw-Hill, 1981.

Morrison, M.L. *Respiratory intensive care* (2nd ed.). Boston: Little, Brown, 1979.

Oral kayexalate causes aspiration pneumonia. *Nurses' Drug Alert,* 1982, 46.

Ryan, A.M. Pneumonia: Aggressive treatment is the key. *RN,* **45**(8), 1982, 44–50.

Zimmerman, G.A., Morris, A.H., and Cengiz, M. Cardiovascular alterations in the adult respiratory distress syndrome. *The American Journal of Medicine,* **73**, 1982, 25–34.

20. Spontaneous Pneumothorax

DEFINITION AND CAUSATIVE FACTORS

Spontaneous pneumothorax occurs when air enters the space between the parietal and visceral pleura. Normally, the intrapleural pressure is less than the atmospheric pressure (760 mm Hg = 0). Quiet breathing causes a change in the intrapleural pressure of between −3 and −5 mm Hg and deep inspiration reduces it to −80 mm Hg. This negative intrapleural pressure is necessary to prevent the lungs from recoiling and losing their expandability. Spontaneous pneumothorax in the client with cancer occurs because of bronchial obstruction or parenchymal lung tissue destruction resulting from malignant tumor invasion or metastasis. The endogenous break in the lung surface allows inspired air to escape into the pleural space causing a positive intrapleural pressure, lung compression, and collapse. Tension pneumothorax with mediastinal shift (Fig. 20-1), compression of the vena cavas and aorta, and cardiac tamponade are the most serious sequelae. Other complications include hemothorax, pleural effusion, and empyema.

Corresponding cancers are lung and metastatic testicular or osteogenic malignancies. Subclavian insertion, proximal gastrectomy, and surgical adrenalectomy are additional causes.

ASSESSMENT DATA

- Sudden sharp, stabbing chest pain
- Acute shortness of breath
- Anxiety, restlessness
- Change in LOC
- Tachycardia, tachypnea
- Decreased or absent breath sounds
- Asymmetrical chest movement
- Hyperresonance on percussion
- Tracheal shift to unaffected side
- Shift of the PMI from fifth ICS, MCL

123

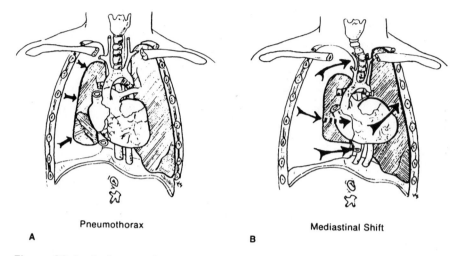

Pneumothorax   Mediastinal Shift

A   **B**

Figure 20-1. A. Pneumothorax. **B**. Mediastinal shift. Note collapse of lung with pneumothorax as air gathers in pleural space. With mediastinal shift, in addition to collapse of the lung, the mediastinal contents are displaced against the unaffected side of chest. Source: Luckman, J., and Sorensen, K.C., 1980, with permission.

NURSING DIAGNOSES	RATIONALE
Ineffective breathing patterns, related to ventilation-perfusion mismatch because of a decrease in lung surface and alveolar function.	*Positive intrapleural pressure causes eventual lung collapse.*

NURSING INTERVENTIONS

Monitoring–Independent

1. Auscultate breath sounds in all lung fields q 2 hr and record onset of diminished or absent sounds.
2. Inspect thorax for symmetry of respiratory movement, use of accessory muscles, and tracheal position q 1 to 2 hr.
3. Assess client for increased respiratory effort, tachypnea, and dyspnea with each contact.
4. Assess client for chest pain with each contact and record location, onset, intensity, and associated factors (increased BP, diaphoresis, nausea and vomiting, SOB, and anxiety).

5. Assess LOC q 2 to 4 hr and record changes in awareness, orientation, and behavior.
6. Auscultate heart sounds in 4 valvular sites q 4 to 8 hr and record onset of gallop or murmur.
7. Inspect for neck vein distention in cm with HOB at 60° q 8 hr.
8. Assess skin color, temperature, moisture, and subcutaneous emphysema q 2 to 4 hr.
9. Palpate peripheral pulses for bilateral quality q 8 hr.
10. Rectal temperature q 6 hr.
11. BP, heart rate, and respirations q 2 hr.
12. Hourly I and O and calculate I/O ratio for fluid balance q 8 and 24 hr.
13. Assess IV site for redness, pain, swelling q 4 to 8 hr.

Monitoring–Interdependent

1. Assess function of chest tube suction.
   Inspect chest tube insertion site for air tightness and all connections for secure fit q 8 hr. Tape with clear adhesive.
   Palpate skin around chest tube and chest wall for subcutaneous emphysema q 8 hr.
   Secure chest tubes so that looping or kinking does not occur and tubing is in descending position (dependent loops obstruct gravity and create back pressure).
   Inspect chest tube and water seal bottle for tidalling (fluctuations that correspond with inspiration–expiration) q 4 to 8 hr.
   Inspect chest tube drainage q 4 to 8 hr for amount and color.
   Inspect degree of bubbling in suction control bottle or compartment and describe as continuous or intermittent, noisy or silent, turbulent or placid q 8 hr (evacuating air creates bubbling).
   Assess pressure gauge or compartment for prescribed suction pressure q 8 hr (usually 20 cm H_2O).
   Note: In this situation, a chest tube should never be clamped. Stripping or milking chest tubes is presently controversial. Unless there is good reason to do so, it is best to omit these practices.
2. Assess laboratory data when available and compare to previous and normal values.
   ABGs pH: 7.35 to 7.45
           P_{O_2}: 75 to 100 torr
           P_{CO_2}: 35 to 45 torr
           HCO_3: 24 to 30 mEq/L
           CO_2 Content: 24 to 30 mEq/L
           O_2 Saturation: 95 to 100%

3. Assess results of serial chest x-rays for lung reexpansion and intrapleural placement of chest tube.

Change–Independent

1. Elevate HOB to 45 to 90° or position of maximum comfort.
2. Humidified O_2 at 2 L/min by nasal cannula or as prescribed by physician.
3. Maintain bedrest and minimize activity with onset of symptoms and for 24 hr after chest tube insertion or as prescribed by physician.
4. Turn unaffected side to back q 2 hr (turning to affected side may kink chest tube and prevent lung reexpansion).
5. Cough and deep breathe q 2 hr.
6. Passive ROME q 4 hr to all major joints alternating with gradual activity schedule.
7. Gradual activity schedule q 4 hr or as prescribed by physician.
8. Back care and massage all bony prominences with lotion q 4 hr.
9. Mouth care using an oral antiseptic q 4 hr if client NPO. Once a day, clean teeth with a mixture of H_2O_2 and baking soda to neutralize oral acid and remove plaque.
10. Force fluids to 150 ml q 1 hr alternating with juice and water.
11. Maintain frequent physical and visual contact with client during acute onset of symptoms and after insertion of chest tube stating time of return before leaving.
12. Reorient to time, place, reason for hospitalization with each contact if client confused or disoriented.
13. Before all procedures, explain purpose and technique using understandable terms.
14. Eliminate all environmental safety hazards. Keep side rails up and pad if client restless or confused, place call light and personal articles within easy reach.
15. Assist client to perform ADLs and maintain judicious independence and control over self and environment within physical limitations.
16. Explain condition and progress to client and family with each contact. Assist them to ask questions and express concerns of the present and the future.
17. Include family members in plan of care and allow them to participate, if mutually beneficial.

Change–Interdependent

1. D5W at KVO or as prescribed by physician.
2. Medicate appropriately for pain and assess effect in 10 to 20 min.

3. Notify physician if:

Chest tube becomes dislodged at insertion site

Increasing dyspnea and restlessness occur *concurrent* with a decrease or increase in bubbling, tidalling, or drainage from chest tube suction. Excessive bubbling in water seal can result from air leak internally in chest or externally in system. Decreased bubbling can result from an occlussion in chest tube, kinking, accidental removal from pleural space, or disconnection of tubing. The bottom line is always the respiratory status of the client. Trouble shoot before notifying physician.

pH less than 7.35 or greater than 7.45

Po_2 less than 70 torr

Pco_2 less than 30 torr or greater than 45 torr

O_2 saturation less than 90%

Chest tube drainage becomes sanguinous (hemothorax), straw colored (pleural effusion), or purulent (empyema)

4. Anticipate physician to prescribe:

Thoracentesis and chest tube insertion with onset of symptoms of pneumothorax

Broad spectrum antibiotics to prevent or eliminate infection

Clamping of chest tube after reexpansion of lung prior to chest tube removal to determine tolerance. (Assess for dyspnea and tension pneumothorax during this period.)

Surgical intervention, if lung does not reexpand after 7 days, to surgically close defect or bronchopleural fistula

Mild analgesia to relieve pain without depressing respirations

Chemotherapy or radiation therapy.

BIBLIOGRAPHY

Bricker, P.L. Chest tubes—The critical points you mustn't forget. *RN*, **43**(11), 1980, 21–26.

Cohen, S. How to work with chest tubes: Programmed instruction. *American Journal of Nursing*, **80**(4), 1980, 685–712.

Corbett, J.V. *Laboratory tests in nursing practice*. Norwalk, Connecticut: Appleton-Century-Crofts, 1982.

Fletcher, B. *Quick reference to critical care nursing*. Philadelphia: J.B. Lippincott, 1983.

Gordon, M. *Manual of nursing diagnosis*. New York: McGraw-Hill, 1982.

Hudak, C.M., Lohr, T., and Gallo, B. *Critical care nursing*. Philadelphia: J.B. Lippincott, 1982.

Kinney, M.R., et al. *A.A.C.N.'s clinical reference for critical care nursing*. New York: McGraw-Hill, 1981.

Luckman, J., and Sorensen, K.C. *Medical-surgical nursing.* Philadelphia: W.B. Saunders, 1980.

Morrison, M.L. *Respiratory intensive care nursing* (2nd ed.). Boston: Little, Brown, 1979.

Perdue, P. Life-threatening respiratory injuries. *RN*, **44**(4), 1981, 27–33.

Woodin, L.M. Your patient with a pneumothorax—A patient in distress. *Nursing 82*, **12**(11), 1982, 50–56.

21. Pleural Effusion

DEFINITION AND CAUSATIVE FACTORS

Pleural effusion is an exudative process in which irritation of the pleural membrane by cancer cells results in an increased production of fluid into the interpleural space. Although direct invasion of the pleural cavity is rare, cancer in the lung can cause obstructed lymphatic drainage and an increased capillary permeability by tumor emboli resulting in pleural fluid accumulation. Normally, 5 to 15 ml of fluid is contained between the visceral and parietal pleura. With as much as 300 ml, lung expansion is compromised, and dyspnea, pain, and compensatory indications of hypoxia develop. Mediastinal shift is a serious complication. Pleural effusion is highly suggestive of extensive intrathoracic cancer, and it may be the first indication of ovarian cancer. Prognosis is ominous, with a 95% death rate within one year. Systemic chemotherapy and intrapleural injections of thio-TEPA or bleomycin are effective treatments.

Corresponding cancers include lymphoma, lung, breast, leukemia, mesothelioma, and metastasis to lung from other primaries. Congestive heart failure, pneumonia, hypoalbuminemia, atelectasis, cirrhosis, pancreatitis, asbestos exposure, superior vena cava syndrome, and irradition are additional causes. Laceration of the subclavian artery during attempts to insert a subclavian catheter is a rare cause.

ASSESSMENT DATA

- Dyspnea
- Pleuritic chest pain—pain on deep inspiration localized to affected side
- Cough
- Tachycardia
- Tachypnea
- Asymmetrical bulging of intercostal spaces

- Dullness on percussion over fluid area
- Decreased fremitus
- Decreased or absent breath sounds depending on severity
- Chest x-ray indications of pleural effusion

NURSING DIAGNOSES	RATIONALE
Ineffective breathing patterns, related to mechanical obstruction to lung inflation, decreasing pulmonary function.	*Lymphoma causes a rupture of the thoracic duct and drainage into the pleural space.*

Associated Nursing Diagnoses

1. Alteration in comfort level, related to acute pain on inspiration, caused by irritation and stretching of pleura.	Pleural fluid accumulation causes pain fiber stimulation.

NURSING INTERVENTIONS

Monitoring–Independent

1. Auscultate breath sounds in all lung fields q 2 to 4 hr and record onset of decreased or absent sounds. (Do not expect to hear a friction rub because fluid separates the pleura.)
2. Inspect thorax for symmetry of respiratory movement, use of accessory muscles, and tracheal position q 2 to 4 hr.
3. Assess client for increased respiratory effort and cough with each contact.
4. Assess client for chest pain with each contact and record location, relationship to inhalation–exhalation, intensity, and associated factors (diaphoresis, increased BP and heart rate, SOB, and anxiety).
5. Assess LOC q 8 hr and record changes in awareness, orientation, and behavior.
6. Auscultate heart sounds in 4 valvular sites q 8 hr and record onset of gallop or murmur.
7. Inspect for neck vein distention in cm with HOB at 60° q 8 hr.
8. Assess skin color, temperature, and moisture q 4 to 8 hr.
9. Palpate peripheral pulses for bilateral quality q 8 hr.

10. BP, heart rate, respirations q 2 to 4 hr.
11. Oral temperature q 4 hr.
12. Accurate I and O and calculate I/O ratio for fluid balance q 8 and 24 hr.
13. Assess IV and subclavian site for redness, pain, and swelling q 4 to 8 hr. (See Chapter 39 for pulmonary complications from TPN.)

Monitoring–Interdependent

1. Assess laboratory data when available and compare to previous and normal values.

   ABGs   pH: 7.35 to 7.45
   Po_2: 75 to 100 torr
   Pco_2: 35 to 45 torr
   HCO_3: 24 to 30 mEq/L
   CO_2 Content: 24 to 30 mEq/L
   BE: ± 2 mEq/L
   O_2 Saturation: 95 to 100%

2. Note results of chest x-ray, expecially subclavian catheter placement.
3. If repeated thoracenteses are performed, assess serum protein levels when available.

   Normal value: 6.0 to 8.4 g/dl

Change–Independent

1. Turn, cough, and deep breathe q 2 hr.
2. Elevate HOB at 45 to 60° or position of maximum comfort.
3. Apply humidified O_2 at 2 L/min by nasal cannula or as prescribed by physician.
4. Bedrest with minimized activity with onset of dyspnea.
5. Back care and massage all bony prominences with lotion q 4 hr.
6. ROME q 4 hr to all major joints alternating with gradual activity schedule if prescribed.
7. Mouth care using oral antiseptic q 4 hr if client NPO. Once a day, clean teeth with a mixture of H_2O_2 and baking soda to neutralize oral acid and remove plaque.
8. Force fluids to 120 ml q 1 hr while awake, if applicable.
9. Eliminate all environmental safety hazards. Keep side rails up and pad if client restless or confused, place call light and personal articles within easy reach.
10. Maintain frequent physical and visual contact during acute phase stating time of return before leaving.

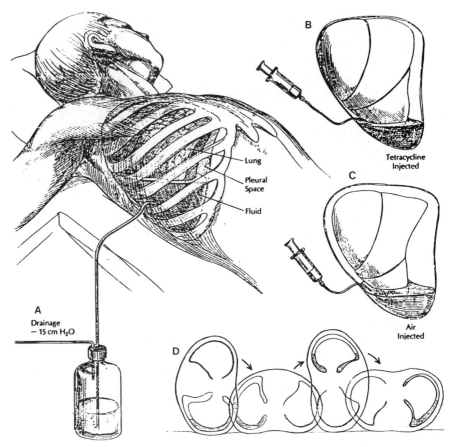

Copyright Carol Donner

Figure 21-1. Sclerosing the pleural space may provide effective palliation for malignant effusions. The fluid is first drained under negative pressure by chest tube (A), and reexpansion of the lung is confirmed radiographically. Next, the sclerosing agent, usually tetracycline, is instilled (B), air is injected to facilitate contact of the tetracycline with all pleural surfaces (C), and the chest tube is clamped. The patient is then rotated to left and right lateral decubitus, prone, and supine positions for 2 to 3 min each (D), and is left in each position for 30 min. Finally, the chest tube is reconnected to negative pressure and left in place for 48 to 72 hr, or until drainage is less than 150 ml/24 hr. Source: Sahn, S.A., 1981, with permission.

11. Explain condition and progress to client and family with each contact. Assist them to ask questions and express concerns of the present and the future.

12. Provide explanation in understandable terms of purpose and technique of procedures.

13. Include family members in plan of care and allow them to participate, if mutually therapeutic.

Change–Interdependent

1. D5W at KVO or as prescribed by physician.
2. Medicate appropriately for pain or anxiety as prescribed and assess effects in 10 to 20 min.
3. Notify physician if:
   Increasing dyspnea with asymmetrical chest expansion, tracheal deviation and/or change in LOC occurs
   pH less than 7.35 or greater than 7.45
   Po_2 less than 70 torr
   Pco_2 less than 30 torr or greater than 45 torr
   O_2 saturation less than 90%
   Severe decrease in serum protein level
   Bleeding, redness, pain, or swelling at subclavian site
4. Anticipate physician to prescribe:
   Thoracentesis and temporary insertion of chest tube to instill sclerosing agent to cause pleural symphysis in order to prevent reoccurrence of pleural effusion. The chest tube remains in place after installation, clamped for 2 hr while the client is rotated in all positions to distribute solution, and removed (Fig. 21-1). Sclerosing solutions include nitrogen mustard, bleomycin, tetracycline, and talc.
   Pleural fluid cytology and protein concentration examination

BIBLIOGRAPHY

Corbett, J.V. *Laboratory tests in nursing practice.* Norwalk, Connecticut: Appleton-Century-Crofts, 1982.
Fentiman, I.S., Rubens, R.D., and Hayward, J.L. The pattern of metastatic disease in patients with pleural effusions secondary to breast cancer. *British Journal of Surgery,* **69,** 1982, 193–194.
Gordon, M. *Manual of nursing diagnosis.* New York: McGraw-Hill, 1982.
Horton, J., and Hill, G.J. *Clinical oncology.* Philadelphia: W.B. Saunders, 1977.
Kinney, M.R., et al. *A.A.C.N.'s clinical reference for critical care nursing.* New York: McGraw-Hill, 1981.
Luckman, J., and Sorensen, K.C. *Medical-surgical nursing—A psychophysiologic approach* (2nd ed.). Philadelphia: W.B. Saunders, 1980.
Morrison, M.L. *Respiratory intensive care nursing* (2nd ed.). Boston: Little, Brown, 1979.
Ostrowski, M.J., and Halsall, G.M. Intracavitary bleomycin in the management of malignant effusions: A multicenter study. *Cancer Treatment Reports,* **66**(11), 1982, 1903–1907.

Portlock, C.S., and Gioffinet, D.R. *Manual of clinical problems in oncology.* Boston: Little, Brown, 1980, Chap. 20.

Sahn, S.A. Pleural manifestations of pulmonary disease. *Hospital Practice,* **16**(3), 1981, 73–89.

Shanes, J.G., Senior, R.M., Stark, D.D., and Baron, R.L. Pleural effusion associated with urinary tract obstruction. *Thorax,* **37,** 1982, 160 (letter).

Wagner, D.W.E. (Ed.). The meaning of pleural effusions. *Emergency Medicine,* **15**(9), 1983, 79–89.

22. Pulmonary Embolism

DEFINITION AND CAUSATIVE FACTORS

Pulmonary thromboembolism originates from large clots formed in the deep veins of the lower extremities or pelvis causing occlusion of a major pulmonary artery. Occlusion can also occur from air (50 ml or more) usually through a central venous line, fat globules released from long bone fractures or soft tissue trauma, or tumor emboli from primary or metastic sites. The obstruction of blood flow to the alveoli causes a reduction of perfused alveoli, bronchoconstriction, and shunting of air to functioning alveoli resulting in atelectasis. Pulmonary infarction, necrosis of pulmonary tissue due to tissue anoxia, has an incidence of less than 10%. With an extensive area of occlusion, pulmonary hypertension, and eventually, cor pulmonale can result. Clients with cancer have a high incidence of pulmonary embolism with a mortality rate of 5%.

Corresponding cancers include pancreas, lung, stomach, colon, and mucinous malignancies. Prolonged immobilization, hypercoagulation, hemoconcentration, debilitation, long bone fractures, soft tissue trauma, and central venous lines are additional causes.

ASSESSMENT DATA

- Pulmonary emboli
  Sudden onset of substernal chest pain
  Dyspnea
  Tachypnea
  Unexplained fever
  Tachycardia
  Change in LOC
  Shock with massive emboli
  Elevated LDH with a normal SGOT
  Respiratory acidosis
  EKG changes

- Fat emboli
  Petechia on anterior chest, shoulders, axilla
  Increased serum lipase
  Fatty sputum
  Symptoms of emboli
- Pulmonary infarction
  Hemoptysis—blood-streaked sputum
  Pleuritic chest pain
  Pleural friction rub
  Symptoms of emboli
- Air emboli
  Disconnected subclavian line with visible air in catheter and symptoms
    of pulmonary emboli
- Atelectasis
  Tracheal shift to affected side
  Dullness on chest percussion
  Diminished or absent breath sounds
- Acute cor pulmonale
  Decreased systolic blood pressure
  Increased diastolic blood pressure
  Increased pulmonary arterial pressure
  Increased central venous pressure
  Palpable right ventricular pulse (at right sternal border, ICS 4 to 5)
  Loud S_2 (pulmonic)
  Gallop rhythm
  Distended neck vein
  Edema
  EKG changes—ST segment depression, T wave inversion in V_{1-3}, new
    S waves in leads I and V_6, Q and T wave inversion in lead III.

NURSING DIAGNOSES	RATIONALE
Impaired gas exchange, related to a reduction of perfused alveoli, bronchoconstriction and collapse of alveolar segments, resulting in hypoxia.	*Air in a subclavian line, fat globules or thrombi cause shunting of air to functioning alveoli and atelectasis of nonfunctioning segments.*

Associated Nursing Diagnoses

1. Alteration of cardiac output, decreased, related to right-sided	Extensive pulmonary occlusion decreases stroke volume and

cardiac involvement, resulting from pulmonary hypertension.

2. Altered comfort level, related to acute pleuritic chest pain and fever.

heart rate, and increase venous return.

Atelectasis, tissue anoxia, and elevated temperature result in the decreased comfort of clients.

NURSING INTERVENTIONS

Monitoring–Independent

1. Auscultate breath sounds in all lung fields q 4 to 8 hr and record onset of diminished, absent, and adventitious sounds.
2. Assess symmetry of chest expansion, use of accessory muscles, depth and ease of respiratory effort with each chest auscultation.
3. Assess for dyspnea, orthopnea, and tachypnea with each client contact.
4. Inspect all sputum for hemoptysis.
5. Assess client for chest pain with each contact and record.
   Location
   Intensity
   Radiation
   Duration
   Aggravating and alleviating factors
   Associated factors—diaphoresis, elevated BP, nausea, vomiting, anxiety
6. Oral temperature q 4 hr.
7. Assess LOC q 4 to 8 hr and record changes in awareness, orientation, and behavior.
8. BP, heart rate, and respirations q 2 hr.
9. Auscultate heart sounds in 4 valvular sites q 4 to 8 hr and record onset of gallop or murmur.
10. Assess neck vein distention in cm with HOB at 60° q 4 to 8 hr.
11. Palpate peripheral pulses for bilateral quality q 8 hr.
12. Assess all dependent areas for edema q 8 hr.
13. Hourly I and O and calculate I/O ratio for fluid balance q 8 and 24 hr.
14. Assess skin color, temperature, moisture, and discolorations q 8 hr.
15. Assess IV site for redness, pain, swelling q 4 to 8 hr.
16. Assess for positive Homan sign in both legs except if deep vein thrombosis has been established. (With phlebothrombosis, this technique can dislodge a clot resulting in embolism.)

Monitoring–Interdependent

1. Assess 12 lead EKG when available for changes indicating pulmonary emboli.

   New incomplete or complete BBB (bundle branch block)

   ST segment depression and T wave inversion in V_{1-3}

   New S waves in lead I and V_6

   Q and T wave inversion in lead III

   Cor pulmonale

   T wave inversion and ST elevation in leads II, III, AVF and V_{1-3}

   Reciprocal changes in lead I

   Deep S waves in V_{5-6} and all limb leads

2. Assess CVP q 2 to 4 hr or as prescribed and compare to previous and normal values: 4 to 8 mm H_2O.

3. Assess laboratory data when available and compare to previous and normal values:

   SGOT: 10 to 40 IU

   LDH: 60 to 120 U/ml

   Serum Lipase: 2 U/ml or less

   ABGs   pH: 7.35 to 7.45

      Po_2: 75 to 100 torr

      Pco_2: 35 to 45 torr

      HCO_3: 24 to 30 mEq/L

      CO_2 Content: 24 to 30 mEq/L

      O_2 Saturation: 95 to 100%

      BE: ± 2 mEq/L

   CBC: Hemoglobin: 13.0 to 18.0 g/dl males

         12.0 to 16.0 g/dl females

      Hematocrit: 45 to 52% males

          37 to 48% females

      RBC: 4.6 to 6.2 × 10^6/mm³ males

        4.2 to 5.4 × 10^6/mm³ females

      MCH: 27 to 32 pg

      MCHC: 32 to 36%

      MCV: 80 to 94 cu microns

      Platelets: 130,000 to 370,000 mm³

      WBC: 4,500 to 11,500/mm³

      Prothrombin Time: control + 4 sec

      Partial Thromboplastin Time: control + 10 sec

      Lee–White Clotting Time: 6 to 17 min

4. Note results of chest x-ray, isotope lung scan, and pulmonary angiography.

5. With anticoagulant therapy assess for bleeding.

   Hemocult all stools

   Observe for hematuria

Hemocult NG tube secretions q 4 hr, if applicable
Inspect oral cavity for bleeding gums
Pad count during menses

Change–Independent

1. Elevate HOB to 60 to 90°.
2. Humidified O_2 at 2 L/min by nasal cannula or as prescribed by physician.
3. Maintain bedrest and minimize activity.
4. Turn, cough, deep breathe q 2 hr.
5. Passive ROME to all major joints *except* in affected leg of confirmed thrombophlebitis q 2 to 4 hr.
6. Back care and massage all bony prominences with lotion q 4 hr.
7. Mouth care using an oral antiseptic q 4 hr if client NPO. Once a day, clean teeth with a mixture of H_2O_2 and baking soda to neutralize oral acid and remove plaque.
8. Force fluids to 120 ml q 1 hr while awake alternating between water and juice EXCEPT if pulmonary hypertension or cor pulmonale has been established. (Fluid overload could be a problem with these conditions.)
9. If air emboli occur due to ingress through a central venous line, turn client on left side with head down (Durant position) to trap air at the top of the right atrium and ventricle and call physician. Prepare equipment for aspiration of air through line.
10. With anticoagulant therapy:
    Mouth care using soft toothbrush or sponge tip applicators and half
       strength H_2O_2
    File fingernails to shortest length
    Remove all jewelry that can abrade skin
    Apply pressure to all venipuncture sites for 10 min
11. Maintain frequent physical and visual contact with client during acute onset of symptoms stating time of return before leaving.
12. Orient client to time, place, and reason for hospitalization with each contact if client confused or disoriented.
13. Eliminate all environmental safety hazards. Keep side rails up and pad if client restless or confused, place call light and personal articles within easy reach.
14. Before all procedures, explain purpose and technique using understandable terms.
15. Explain condition and progress to client and family with each contact. Assist them to ask questions and express concerns of the present and the future.

16. Include family members in plan of care and allow them to participate, if mutually therapeutic.

Change–Interdependent

1. D5W at KVO or as prescribed by physician.
2. Medicate appropriately for pain or anxiety and assess effect in 10 to 20 min.
3. Notify physician if:
     Sudden onset of chest pain occurs
     SOB and tachypnea with EKG changes occur
     Hemoptysis occurs with unexplained temperature elevation
     Palpable right ventricular pulse at right sternal border, 4th ICS occurs with neck vein distention (cor pulmonale)
     Petechia occurs on chest or shoulders with SOB
     Lee–White clotting time greater or less than 25 to 35 min (therapeutic range with anticoagulation therapy)
     Partial thromboplastin time greater or less than (50 to 80S)/(29 to 35S) −2 to 2.5 times normal
     CVP greater than 8 cm H_2O
     pH less than 7.35
     Po_2 less than 75 torr
     Pco_2 greater than 45 torr (uncompensated)
4. Anticipate the physician to prescribe:
     Dextran 40 mg IV to increase pulmonary blood flow
     Streptokinase or urokinase to promote thrombolysis
     Ligation of inferior vena cava or insertion of vena cava umbrella with severe or repeated thromboemboli
     Mechanical ventilation with PEEP with severe respiratory distress
     Tagamet to prevent stress ulcer formation

BIBLIOGRAPHY

Burns, N. *Nursing and cancer.* Philadelphia: W.B. Saunders, 1982.
Corbott, J.V. *Laboratory tests in nursing practice.* Norwalk, Connecticut: Appleton-Century-Crofts, 1982.
Fletcher, B. *Quick reference to critical care nursing.* Philadelphia: J.B. Lippincott, 1983.
Gordon, M. *Manual of nursing diagnosis.* New York: McGraw-Hill, 1982.
Harvey, A.M., Johns, R.J., McKusick, V.A., Owens, A.H., Jr., and Ross, R.S. *The principles and practice of medicine* (20th ed.). New York: Appleton–Century-Crofts, 1980.

Keefer, C.S., and Wilkins, R.W. *Medicine—Essentials of clinical practice.* Boston: Little, Brown, 1970.

Kinney, M.R., et al. *A.A.C.N.'s clinical reference for critical care nursing.* New York: McGraw-Hill, 1981.

Lewis, S.M., and Collier, I.C. *Medical-surgical nursing: Assessment and management of clinical problems.* New York: McGraw-Hill, 1983.

Lyon, L.J. *Basic electrocardiography handbook.* New York: Van Nostrand Reinhold, 1977.

Marriott, H.J.L. *Practical electrocardiography* (6th ed.). Baltimore: Williams and Wilkins, 1977.

Turnbull, A.D. Thoracic emergencies—Pulmonary embolism. In R.C. Hickey (Ed.), *Current problems in cancer* (Vol. 4, No. 3.). Chicago: Year Book Medical, 1979, pp. 57–59.

23. Radiation Pneumonitis

DEFINITION AND CAUSATIVE FACTORS

Radiation pneumonitis is an acute inflammatory response of lung tissue to radiation of the chest. Pathophysiologic changes in the pulmonary system include: alveolar degeneration, fibrin deposition, and hyaline membrane formation in the alveolar spaces resulting in alveolar fibrosis. With moderate radiation doses (100 to 500 Ret), these changes are reversible, but permanent damage may occur with larger amounts of radiation (500 to 800 Ret). The incidence of radiation pneumonitis is less than 5%, but the risk increases to 33% with irradiation to the chest wall for bronchogenic and lung malignancies, and Hodgkin disease. Chemotherapeutic agents, as a contributing factor, include actinomycin D, Adriamycin, busulfan, and bleomycin. Usually the client is asymptomatic, but an onset of symptoms can occur months or years later. Fatality can occur if 75% or more of the lung is involved. Dyspnea is the significant manifestation of radiation pneumonitis.

Corresponding cancers include bronchogenic, lung, and Hodgkin. Sudden cessation of prednisone in the second or fourth cycles of MOPP protocol is an additional cause.

ASSESSMENT DATA

- Dyspnea
- Dry, hacking cough
- Fever
- Cyanosis
- Tachypnea
- Respiratory failure
- X-ray showing blurring of pulmonary markings, dense opacifications
- Previous radiation therapy and dose
- Previous or subsequent chemotherapeutic agents

NURSING DIAGNOSES	RATIONALE
Impaired gas exchange, related to alveolar wall damage preventing the diffusion of O₂ and CO₂.	*Radiation to the chest wall causes alveolar degeneration and hyaline membrane formation followed by fibrosis. Certain chemotherapeutic drugs cause diffuse pulmonary fibrosis.*

NURSING INTERVENTIONS

Monitoring–Independent

1. Auscultate breath sounds in all lung fields q 2 to 4 hr after each radiation treatment and record onset of adventitious sounds or pleural friction rubs.
2. Assess client for dyspnea, tachypnea, and cough with each contact.
3. Assess use of accessory muscles, respiratory effort, and symmetry of chest expansion q 2 to 4 hr.
4. Rectal temperature q 4 hr.
5. Inspect all sputum for hemoptysis.
6. Assess LOC q 4 to 8 hr and record changes in awareness, orientation, and behavior.
7. Assess skin color, temperature, and moisture q 4 to 8 hr.
8. BP, heart rate, respirations q 4 hr.
9. Auscultate heart sounds at 4 valvular sites q 8 hr.
10. Palpate peripheral pulses for bilateral quality q 8 hr.
11. Assess IV site for redness, swelling, and pain q 8 hr.

Monitoring–Interdependent

1. Assess laboratory data when available and compare to previous and normal values.
   ABGs   pH: 7.35 to 7.45
           Po_2: 75 to 100 torr
           Pco_2: 35 to 45 torr
           HCO_3: 24 to 30 mEq/L
           CO_2 Content: 24 to 30 mEq/L
           BE: ± 2 mEq/L
           O_2 Saturation: 95 to 100%

2. Assess results of serial chest x-rays for indication of fibrosis.
3. Assess history for previous radiation therapy. Include time, dose, and volume of lung irradiated.
4. Assess history for previous chemotherapy. Include name of agent(s), dose, and number of treatments.

Change–Independent

1. Elevate HOB at 60 to 90°.
2. Maintain bedrest with minimized activity with onset of dyspnea.
3. Apply humidified O_2 at 2 L/min by nasal cannula or as prescribed by physician.
4. Turn, cough, deep breathe q 2 hr while on bedrest.
5. Mouth care using an oral antiseptic q 4 hr. Once a day, clean teeth with a mixture of H_2O_2 and baking soda to neutralize oral acid and remove plaque.
6. Offer fluids q hr alternating between water and juice of choice.
7. Passive ROME q 4 hr to all major joints while on bedrest, progressing to active ROME q 4 hr.
8. Back care and massage all bony prominences with lotion q 4 hr, avoiding radiation field.
9. Isolate client from others (family, staff, clients) with any infectious process.
10. Eliminate all irritating inhalants from environment.
    Strong cleaning solutions
    Tobacco smoke (visitor and client)
    Heavy scents in personal toiletries
    Aerosols
11. Ambulate with graduated activity schedule or as prescribed by physician.
12. Before all procedures, explain purpose and technique in understandable terms.
13. Reorient to time, place, reason for hospitalization with each contact if client confused or disoriented.
14. Explain condition and progress to client and family with each contact. Assist them to ask questions and express concerns of the present and future.
15. Include family members in plan of care and allow them to participate, if mutually beneficial.
16. Reinforce respiratory rehabilitation therapy if applicable with client and family.
    Diaphragmatic breathing exercises

Pursed lip breathing exercises
IPPB (may be contraindicated)
Incentive spirometry
(Vibration and postural drainage are contraindicated.)

Change–Interdependent

1. D5W at KVO or as prescribed by physician if acute respiratory distress develops.
2. Medicate appropriately for pain as prescribed and assess effect in 10 to 20 min.
3. Notify physician if:
   Friction rub develops
   pH less than 7.35
   P_{O_2} less than 70 torr
   P_{O_2} greater than 45 torr (uncompensated)
   O_2 saturation less than 90%
   Severe dyspnea, respiratory arrest occurs
   Rectal temperature greater than 102° F
4. Anticipate the physician to prescribe:
   Broad spectrum antibiotics to eliminate risks of secondary infections
   Bronchodilators to enhance oxygen delivery
   Prednisone with onset of dyspnea—60 to 100 mg/24 hr
   Discontinuation or change in radiation and/or chemotherapy treatment

BIBLIOGRAPHY

Canellos, G.P., Cohen, G., and Posner, M. Pulmonary emergencies in neoplastic disease. In J. Yarbro and R. Bornstein (Eds.), *Oncologic emergencies*. New York: Grune and Stratton, 1981, pp. 310–313.
Corbett, J.V. *Laboratory tests in nursing practice*. Norwalk, Connecticut: Appleton-Century-Crofts, 1982.
Gordon, M. *Manual of nursing diagnosis*. New York: McGraw-Hill, 1982.
Horton, J., and Hill, G.J. *Clinical oncology*. Philadelphia: W.B. Saunders, 1977.
Kelly, P.P., and Tinsley, C. Planning care for the patient receiving external radiation. *American Journal of Nursing*, 81(2), 1981, 338–342.
Yasko, J.M. Care of the patient receiving radiation therapy. *Nursing Clinics of North America*, 17(4), 1982, 631–648.

PART IV
IMMUNITY

24. Neutropenic and Nonneutropenic Sepsis

DEFINITION AND CAUSATIVE FACTORS

Sepsis and septic shock are conditions caused by gram-negative bacteremia. As with other types of shock, septic shock (Table 24-1) causes massive vasodilatation incurring a deficient circulating blood volume, cardiac output (Fig. 24-1) and tissue perfusion. Cellular hypoxia and acidosis are the devastating end results. Gram-negative organisms produce endotoxins that interfere with the temperature regulatory center in the hypothalamus by elevating the body temperature, damage the endothelium of capillaries causing microthrombi and increased capillary permeability, activate kinins and histamines causing vasodilatation, activate clotting factor XII initiating disseminated intravascular coagulation (Chapter 11), and lyse RBCs producing microhemorrhages throughout the body. The initial symptoms of septic shock occur earlier than other types of shock and classically consist of fever, widening pulse pressure, change in LOC and behavior, and flushed, warm, dry skin. Septic shock is more difficult to treat and has a mortality rate of 60 to 80%.

Among neutropenic clients (polymorphonuclear neutropil count less than 500/cu mm or 10%; normal count is 62%), gram-negative sepsis is the most common cause of death. Neutropenia results from chemotherapy with cytotoxic drugs, radiation, and bone marrow replacement by cancer cells. Nonneutropenic clients are those with normal or elevated PMN counts but develop sepsis because of other risk factors. Complications of septic shock include vascular collapse, shock lung (adult respiratory distress syndrome), renal failure, CHF, cardiac arrhythmias, coma, DIC, and viral and fungal infections.

Corresponding cancers include leukemia, lymphoma, and all cancers treated with cytotoxic chemotherapy and/or radiation for neutropenic

TABLE 24-1. STAGES OF SEPTIC SHOCK

Pathophysiology	Signs and Symptoms
Hyperdynamic stage (warm shock, pink shock) **(Best chance of survival)** Body reacting to invading bacteria: heart and lungs work to keep up with raised need for O_2. Closing of precapillary sphincters leaves arterioles dilated, especially in skin and kidneys; this arteriovenous shunting (with alkalosis) lowers Po_2 and circulating fluid. The 60% of body fluid normally present in the capillary bed is beginning to stay there and be unavailable. Cell metabolism is impaired.	Mental confusion (usually first sign) Chills and fever (usually) Skin flushed, warm Blood pressure normal or slightly ↓ Tachycardia Tachypnea ↓ Po_2 (despite O_2 administration) Urine output normal to slightly ↑
Normodynamic stage (cool shock) **(Lasts only a few hours)** Body reacting to endotoxins released by dying bacteria. Anoxia in capillary bed, capillary leakage, third spacing of fluid, less venous return. Congestion and relative hypovolemia worsen. Compensation is at work: Proteins now concentrated in the circulation begin drawing fluid back from third spaces, and catecholamines constrict blood vessels, lowering urine output, increasing cardiac rate and force, and causing dry mouth.	Cool skin Peripheral edema Tachycardia Blood pressure normal or slightly ↓ Hyperventilation Pulmonary congestion Progressive hypoxemia Oliguria Thirst
Hypodynamic stage (cold shock) **(Most dangerous stage)** Classic "shock." Blood goes into capillaries but can't get out; pronounced capillary leakage, caused by bacterial endotoxins and proteolytic enzymes from damaged cells, increases anaerobic metabolism. This worsens metabolic acidosis, fluid loss into tissues, and hypovolemia. Vasoconstriction gives way to vasodilation followed by circulatory collapse. Microthrombi in leaking capillaries may lead to DIC, acute respiratory distress syndrome to respiratory failure, renal ischemia to renal failure and necrosis. Prognosis is poor.	Cold, clammy skin Tachycardia, thready pulse Severe hypotension High CVP, PWP Respiratory failure Profound hypoxemia Metabolic acidosis Severe oliguria or anuria

(Source: from Lamb, L.S. 1982, with permission.)

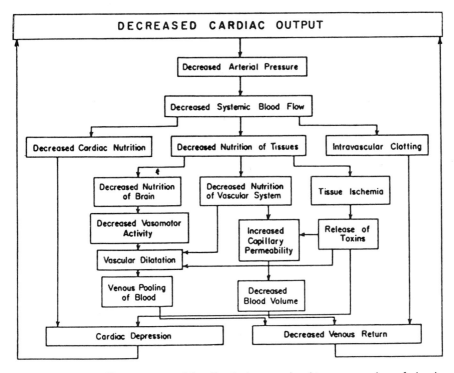

Figure 24-1. Different types of feedback that can lead to progression of shock. Source: Guyton, A.C., 1976, with permission.

sepsis; and solid tumors, GI, and GU tumors for nonneutropenic sepsis. Intrusive body catheters, severe debilitation, surgery, chronic liver disease, and infection related to bacteria, fungi, viruses, and parasites are additional causes.

ASSESSMENT DATA (TABLE 24-2)

- WBC less than $1,000/mm^3$ or greater than $10,000/mm^3$
- Oral temperature elevation of 100.2° F or more
- Flushed, warm, dry skin
- Widening pulse pressure followed by a decreased blood pressure
- Developing confusion, apprehension, lethargy
- Thrombocytopenia
- Prolonged PT and PTT

- Positive blood cultures for gram-negative bacteria
    E. coli
    P. aeruginosa
    Klebsiella
    Bacterioides

NURSING DIAGNOSES	RATIONALE
Fluid volume deficit, related to deficient blood volume due to generalized vasodilatation and pooling caused by the toxic effect of gram-negative bacteremia.	*Endotoxins increase capillary permeability and activate kinins and histamines causing vasodilatation.*

Associated Nursing Diagnoses

1. Alteration in cardiac output, decreased, related to decreased venous return, due to vasodilatation and pooling.

   Capillary leakage and third spacing of fluid decreases venous return causing hypovolemia.

2. Impaired gas exchange, related to a lack of RBC availability for alveolar and cellular O_2 and CO_2 exchange.

   Lysis of RBCs due to activation of clotting factor XII.

3. Impairment of urinary elimination, related to a decreased perfusion to the kidney, causing a decreased glomular filtration rate and cellular damage.

   Hypovolemia causes insufficient renal arterial pressure necessary to maintain glomerular filtration.

4. Alteration in tissue perfusion related to cerebral hypoxia, causing a change in LOC and behavior.

   Anaerobic metabolism is increased which worsens metabolic acidosis. Endotoxins damage endothelium causing microthrombi.

NURSING INTERVENTIONS

Monitoring–Independent

1. Oral temperature q 4 hr.
2. BP, heart rate, respirations q 2 hr. Document pulse pressure with each BP reading. ·

3. Assess LOC q 8 hr and document changes in awareness, orientation, and behavior.
4. Assess skin color, temperature, moisture, discolorations (petechia, bruising) q 4 to 8 hr.
5. Auscultate breath sounds in all lung fields, symmetry of chest expansion, use of accessory muscles q 8 hr, and record onset of adventitious sounds.
6. Auscultate heart sounds at 4 valvular sites q 8 hr and record onset of gallop or murmur.
7. Palpate peripheral pulses for bilateral quality q 8 hr.
8. Assess all dependent areas for edema q 8 hr.
9. Hourly I and O and calculate I/O ratio for fluid balance q 8 and 24 hr.
10. Hemocult all stools and emesis.
11. Urine specific gravity qd.
12. Auscultate bowel sounds in 4 quadrants and assess abdomen for rigidity and tenderness q 8 hr.
13. Weigh daily and compare weight to previous day. (1 kg wt gain = 1000 ml retention, a critical assessment if client in renal failure.)
14. Assess IV site for redness, swelling, or pain q 4 to 8 hr.

Monitoring–Interdependent

1. Pulmonary artery pressure q 1 hr and compare to previous and normal value.
   Systolic: 20 to 30 torr
   Diastolic: 8 to 15 torr
2. *Or* central venous pressure q 1 hr and compare to previous and normal value.
   CVP: 0 to 5 mm Hg
   CVP: 4 to 8 cm H_2O
3. Pulmonary capillary wedge pressure q 4 hr or as prescribed by physician, and compare to previous and normal value: 4 to 12 torr, 18 maximum.
4. Cardiac output and index q 4 hr or as prescribed by physician, and compare to previous and normal values.
   Cardiac output: 4 to 8 L/min
   Cardiac index: 3.5 ± 0.7 L/min/m^2
5. Assess oral cavity for white patches indicating fungal superimposed infection and vagina for discharge.
6. Obtain cultures of suspected origin(s) of sepsis or sputum, oral, vaginal, wound, blood, urine, catheters.

7. Assess laboratory data when available and compare to previous and normal values.

   WBC: 4,500 to 11,500/mm³
   Platelet Count: 130,000 to 370,000 mm³
   Prothrombin Time: control plus 4 sec
   Partial Thromboplastin Time: control plus 10 sec

TABLE 24-2. DIAGNOSTIC STUDY ABNORMALITIES IN SHOCK SYNDROME

Diagnostic Study	Abnormal Finding	Significance of Abnormality
Blood		
RBCs hematocrit, hemoglobin	Normal	Remains within normal limits in shock due to relative hypovolemia and pump failure and in hemorrhagic shock prior to fluid resuscitation.
	Decreased	Decreased in hemorrhagic shock following fluid resuscitation when fluids other than blood are used.
	Increased	Increased in nonhemorrhagic shock due to actual hypovolemia because the fluid lost does not contain erythrocytes.
WBC with differential	Leukopenia	Occurs in severe shock, especially when it is due to gram-negative sepsis.
	Leukocytosis with increased neutrophils	Common in all forms of shock, especially hemorrhagic shock. Neutrophils increase in response to tissue injury.
Erythrocyte sedimentation rate	Increased	Nonspecific; increases in response to tissue injury.
BUN	Increased	Usually indicates impaired kidney function due to hypoperfusion.
Serum creatinine	Increased	Usually indicates impaired kidney function due to hypoperfusion. A more sensitive indicator of renal function than BUN.
Blood sugar	Increased	Occurs in early shock due to release of liver glycogen stores in response to catecholamines.
	Decreased	As shock progresses, glycogen stores are depleted and hepatocellular dysfunction may occur.

TABLE 24-2. (Continued)

Diagnostic Study	Abnormal Finding	Significance of Abnormality
Blood		
Arterial blood gases	Respiratory alkalosis	Occurs early in shock secondary to hyperventilation
	Metabolic acidosis	Occurs when organic acids, such as lactic acid, accumulate in the blood from anaerobic metabolism.
Blood cultures	Growth of one organism (usually)	Gram-negative organisms are most frequently seen in patients who are in septic shock.
Serum Electrolytes:		
Sodium	Increased	Occurs when shock is due to gastrointestinal fluid loss or diabetes insipidus. Also occurs during the diuretic phase of acute tubular necrosis.
	Decreased	May occur iatrogenically when excess hypotonic fluid is administered following a fluid loss.
Potassium	Increased	Occurs when cellular death liberates intracellular potassium. Also occurs in acute renal failure, following RBC hemolysis in transfusion reactions, and when acidosis is present.
	Decreased	May occur when vomiting or excessive gastric suctioning is the cause of shock.
Calcium	Decreased	Sometimes occurs following rapid infusion of large amounts of citrated blood. Also occurs secondary to the respiratory alkalosis of early shock.
	Increased	Occurs secondary to lactic acidosis, which permits increased ionization of calcium.
Urine		
Specific gravity	Increased	Occurs secondary to the action of ADH.
	Fixed at 1.010	Occurs in acute tubular necrosis.

(Source: from Lewis S.M. and Collier, I.C., 1983, with permission.)

Fibrinogen: 200 to 500 mg/dl
Hemoglobin: 13.0 to 18.0 g/dl males
               12.0 to 16.0 g/dl females
Hematocrit: 45 to 52% males
               37 to 48% females
ABGs: pH: 7.35 to 7.45
      Po_2: 75 to 100 torr
      Pco_2: 35 to 45 torr
      HCO_3: 24 to 30 mEq/L
      BE: ± 2 mEq/L
      CO_2 Content: 24 to 30 mEq/L
BUN: 8 to 25 mg/dl (especially if renal failure suspected or nephrotoxic antibiotic used)
Creatinine: 0.6 to 1.5 mg/dl
Serum Sodium: 135 to 145 mEq/L
Serum Chloride: 100 to 106 mEq/L
Serum Potassium: 3.5 to 5.0 mEq/L
Serum Calcium: 8.5 to 10.5 mg/dl

Change–Independent

1. Bedrest and minimize activity.
2. Oral care using soft toothbrush with half strength H_2O_2 or other special oral agents q 4 hr. Once a day, clean teeth with a mixture of H_2O_2 and baking soda to neutralize oral acid and remove plaque.
3. O_2 at 2L/min by nasal cannula or as prescribed by physician.
4. Apply pressure to all venipunctures for 10 min or until bleeding stops. Coordinate all laboratory work so that venipunctures are minimized.
5. Change subclavian dressing q 48 hr or according to protocol if Swan–Ganz, TPN or central venous catheter in place.
6. Turn q 2 hr and back care with friction massage to all bony prominences q 4 hr.
7. Cough and deep breathe q 2 hr if client not on ventilator or suction q 1 hr using hyperinflation and hyperoxygenation techniques with ventilator.
8. Passive ROME to all extremities using caution with arm used for intraarterial pressure line.
9. File fingernails to shortest length and brush clean qd.
10. Explain condition and progress to client and family with each contact. Assist them to ask questions and express concerns for the present and the future.
11. Reorient to time, place, reason for hospitalization with each contact if client confused or disoriented.

12. Make frequent physical and visual contact with client during acute phase stating time of return before leaving.
13. Eliminate all environmental safety hazards; keep side rails up and pad if client restless and disoriented.
14. Include family members in plan of care and allow them to participate; if mutually therapeutic.

Change–Interdependent

1. D5W at KVO or as prescribed by physician.
2. Notify physician if:
    WBC less than 1,000/mm^3
    Pulmonary artery diastolic pressure less than 8 or greater than 20 torr
    CVP less than 4 or greater than 10 cm H_2O
    Pulmonary wedge pressure less than 4 or greater than 18 torr
    Cardiac index less than 4 or greater than 8 L/min
    Systolic blood pressure less than 90 mm Hg
    Oral temperature greater than 101.0° F and progressively widening pulse pressure with change in LOC and urinary output less than 30 ml/hr
    Platelet count less than 50,000 mm^3
    Prolonged PT and PTT
    Hemoglobin less than 10 g/dl
    Hematocrit less than 30%
    Serum calcium less than 8 mg/dl
    Serum potassium greater than 6.0 mEq/L
    Nurse suspects signs or symptoms of early sepsis
    Cultures positive for pathogens and current antibiotic therapy not sensitive
3. Anticipate physician to prescribe:
    Stop cytotoxic chemotherapy with WBC less than 1,000 mm^3
    Antibiotic therapy for suspected signs and symptoms of early sepsis
    Aggressive IV antibiotic therapy with cephalosporins and aminoglycosides (both nephrotoxic and ototoxic) to eliminate bacterial agent(s)
    Blood cultures $\times$3 with oral temperature greater than 101°F to isolate organism
    Dexamethasone: 3 mg/kg to stabilize capillary membrane and suppress inflammatory reaction
    Hemodynamic monitoring to assess vascular and intercardiac pressures in order to evaluate fluid and volume status
    Mechanical ventilation with endotracheal tube to maintain Po_2 at 75 to 100 torr and prevent ARDS

Hypothermia blanket to reduce temperature

Fluid challenge of 200 ml/hr with Ringer's lactate or 10% dextran, or according to CVP or hemodynamic monitoring

Digoxin to increase force of myocardial contractility

Dopamine to strengthen myocardial contractility and cause peripheral vasoconstriction which increases pressure and perfusion

Isuprel to decrease venous pooling and increase cardiac contractility and rate

Levophed to cause vasoconstriction and increase cardiac contractility and rate

(These drugs are usually used in combinations.)

WBC transfusions of family member with HLA lymphocyte grade A matches with WBC less than 500/mm^3

NaHCO$_3$ to correct acidosis

Mycostatin mouthwash and swallow to treat or prevent fungal infections

Platelet transfusions if platelet count less than 20,000 mm^3

Total parenteral nutrition using amino acid and fatty acid solutions (Chapter 39)

Dialysis if BUN and creatinine critically elevated

BIBLIOGRAPHY

Brunkhorst, L., Walden, J., Castro, R., and Hayakawa, K. Management of the septic patient with leukemia who requires ventilatory assistance. *Heart and Lung,* **12**(6), 1983, 636–642.

Corbett, J.V. *Laboratory tests in nursing practice.* Norwalk, Connecticut: Appleton-Century-Crofts, 1982.

Gordon, M. *Manual of nursing diagnosis.* New York: McGraw-Hill, 1982.

Guyton, A.C. *Textbook of medical physiology* (6th ed.). Philadelphia: W.B. Saunders, 1981.

Hall, K.V. Detecting septic shock before it's too late. *RN* **43**(9), 1981, 29–32.

Harvey, A.M., Johns, R.J., McKusick, V.A., Owens, A.H., Jr., and Ross, R.S. *The principles and practice of medicine* (20th ed.). New York: Appleton-Century-Crofts, 1980.

Horton, J., and Hill, G.J. *Clinical oncology.* Philadelphia: W.B. Saunders, 1977.

Hudak, C.M., Lohr, T., and Gallo, B. *Critical Care Nursing.* Philadelphia: J.B. Lippincott, 1982.

Johanson, B.C., et al. *Standards for critical care.* St. Louis: C.V. Mosby, 1981.

Kaye, W. Catheter and infusion-related sepsis: The nature of the problem and its prevention. *Heart and Lung,* **11**(3), 1982, 221–227.

Kinney, M.R., et al. *A.A.C.N.'s clinical reference for critical care nursing.* New York: McGraw-Hill, 1981.

Lamb, L.S. Think you know septic shock? *Nursing 82,* **12**(1), 1982, 34–43.

Lewis, S.M., and Collier, I.C. *Medical-surgical nursing: Assessment and management of clinical problems.* New York: McGraw-Hill, 1983.

Riben, P.D., et al. Reduction in mortality from gram-negative sepsis in neutropenic patients receiving trimethoprim/sulfamethoxazole therapy. *Cancer,* **51,** 1983, 1587–1592.

Rosenthal, S.N., and Bennett, J.M. *Practical cancer chemotherapy.* New York: Medical Examination, 1981.

Smith, D.L. Septic shock. *Topics in Emergency Medicine,* **5**(2), 1983, 34–39.

Yasko, J.M. Septic shock. In J.M. Yasko (ed.), *Guidelines for cancer care—Symptom management.* Virginia: Reston, 1983, pp. 347–352.

25. Chemotherapy Related Anaphylaxis

DEFINITION AND CAUSATIVE FACTORS

Anaphylaxis in the client with cancer is a type I hypersensitivity reaction to a chemotherapeutic agent which becomes the antigen. Type I hypersensitivity reactions involve the antibody IgE, mast cells, basophils, and sensitization of the host by previous exposure to the antigen. Mast cells are located in connective tissue, and basophils function in nonspecific immunologic reactions in the general circulation. In people who are sensitized, the mast cell will contain the particular antibody to react with the antigen, and the B-lymphocyte will produce more IgE immunoglobulins when additional antigens are introduced. Because the antigen, the chemotherapeutic agent, is administered intravenously, the distribution of the antigen is systemic, and anaphylaxis results.

Antigen (chemotherapeutic agent)→ IgE immunoglobulins produced→ Bind to mast cells in connective tissue→ Mast cell degradation→ ↓cAMP→ Systemic reaction

Mast cell degradation causes a decreased production of cyclic adenosine monophosphate (cAMP). This is necessary to inhibit mediator release, factors that initiate the effect of anaphylaxis, and regulators, agents that neutralize the effects initiated by mediators (Table 25-1). Anaphylaxis occurs when the body mediators outgain the regulatory agents causing intercompartmental fluid shift from the extracellular space to the intercellular space, vasodilatation, bronchial constriction, smooth muscle contraction, and pain. Anaphylactic shock has a high mortality rate, and it occurs more frequently with L-asparaginase (6 to 43%), Cisplatin (1 to 20%), topical Mechlorethamine (nitrogen mustard), Melphalan (Alkeran), and Teniposide (VM-26).

Corresponding cancers include all those treated with chemotherapy.

TABLE 25-1. MEDIATORS AND REGULATORY AGENTS OF ANAPHYLAXIS

Mediators	Regulatory Agent
Histamine	*Eosinophil chemotactic factor*
Smooth muscle contraction	Releases 3 enzymes
Vascular permeability increased	*Histaminase:* Degrades histamine
Mucous secretion increased	*Sulphatase B:* Disposes of slow-reacting substance
Slow-reacting substance	*Phospholipid D:* Destroys platelet activating factor
Visceral smooth muscle spasms	
Vascular permeability increased	
Platelet activating factor	
Aggregation of platelets	
Degranulation of platelets	
Kinins	
Vasodilatation	
Hypotension	
Smooth muscle contraction	
Bronchial constriction	
GI motility increased	
Heart rate increased	
Cardiac output increased	
Nerve endings of skin irritated	
Prostaglandins	
Smooth muscle contraction (stomach and intestines)	
Antagonizes lipolyses induced by epinephrine	
Hypotension (in hypertensive humans)	

ASSESSSMENT DATA

- Shortness of breath
- Wheezing, stridor
- Puffy face and/or dependent edema
- Urticaria
- Itching skin
- Dizziness
- Hypotension
- Abdominal cramps

- Chest pain
- Decreased plasma volume in circulation
- Increased blood viscosity
- Decreased pulse volume
- Weakness of extremities
- Vomiting
- Weight gain
- Cyanosis

NURSING DIAGNOSES	RATIONALE
Fluid volume deficit, related to an adverse response to chemotherapy, resulting in a shift of fluid from extravascular compartments to intracellular compartments.	*Failure of body regulatory agents— eosinophil chemotactic factor, histaminase, sulphatase B, and phospholipid D—resulting in vasoconstriction and hypovolemia.*

Associated Nursing Diagnoses

1. Ineffective breathing pattern, related to wheezing, shortness of breath, and cyanosis, resulting in bronchoconstriction.	Systemic body reaction caused by the release of mediator agents: histamine, slow-reacting substance, platelet activating factor, kinins, and prostoglandins.
2. Altered comfort level, related to urticaria, itching, abdominal cramps and acute chest pain, resulting from a systemic hypersensitivity reaction.	Smooth muscle contraction caused by the release of mediator agents: histamine, slow-reacting substance, kinins, and prostaglandins.

NURSING INTERVENTIONS

Monitoring–Independent

1. BP, heart rate q 5 to 15 min until stable with onset of symptoms, q 1 hr during chemotherapy, and q 1 to 2 hr after hypotensive episode and/or chemotherapy administration.
2. Assess respiratory rate, depth, and use of accessory muscles q 5 to 15 min until stable with onset of symptoms.
3. Assess for dyspnea, cyanosis, and wheezing q 5 to 15 min until stable with onset of symptoms, q 1 hr during chemotherapy (initial or subsequent doses) and q 4 hr after chemotherapy.
4. Rectal temperature q 1 hr during and after chemotherapy ×4.
5. Assess for chest pain and abdominal cramps using objective and subjective data q 15 to 30 min during chemotherapy and q 4 hr after chemotherapy.
6. Assess skin for urticaria and itching, record changes in size and intensity q 30 min during chemotherapy and q 2–4 hr after chemotherapy.
7. Auscultate breath sounds in all lung fields q 2 hr and record onset of rales and rhonchi during chemotherapy and q 4 to 8 hr after chemotherapy.

8. Assess face, eyelids, and earlobes for edema q 1 hr with onset of symptoms.
9. Assess LOC q 8 hr and record changes in awareness, orientation, and behavior.
10. Measure ankles and abdominal girth using predetermined landmarks q 8 hr and compare to previous measurements.
11. Weigh q AM before breakfast and compare to previous measurements.
12. Hemocult all stools and emesis.
13. Accurate I and O, calculate I/O ratio for fluid balance q 8 and 24 hr.
14. Auscultate heart sounds in 4 valvular sites q 8 hr and record onset of extra heart sounds or changes in rhythm.
15. Auscultate bowel sounds in 4 quadrants and record changes in frequency.

Monitoring–Interdependent

1. Inspect skin test for chemotherapy sensitivity as prescribed in 5 to 20 min. A drop of the chemotherapeutic agent is placed on the skin and pricked. The development of a wheal greater than 3 mm wide indicates that the client is sensitized or atopic, and therefore at risk for anaphylaxis.
2. Assess results of laboratory data when available and compare to previous and normal values.
   Hemoglobin: 13.0 to 18.0 g/dl males
                12.0 to 16.0 g/dl females
   Hematocrit: 45 to 52% males
                37 to 48% females
   ABGs pH: 7.35 to 7.45
          Po_2: 75 to 100 torr
          Pco_2: 35 to 45 torr
          HCO_3: 24 to 30 mEq/L
          O_2 Saturation: 95 to 100%
          CO_2 Content: 24 to 30 mEq/L
   IgE Antibody: less than 1 mg/dl

Change–Independent

1. Discontinue chemotherapy stat with systolic BP 90 torr or less and onset of dyspnea, wheezing, or urticaria.
2. Apply O_2 at 2 L/min by nasal cannula
3. IV 0.9% saline or D5W at 30 ml/hr or as prescribed.
4. Apply ice collar to neck with indications of nausea or vomiting.

5. Maintain on bedrest during chemotherapy with HOB at 30 to 60°, with onset of symptoms HOB flat unless contraindicated by respiratory distress.
6. Offer 120 ml clear liquids po q 2 hr while awake if appropriate.
7. Bathe client with cool baking soda bath when condition stable.
8. Turn, cough, deep breathe q 2 hr. while on bedrest.
9. Passive ROME to all extremities (except IV arm) q 4 hr.
10. Mouth care using $\frac{1}{2}$ strength H_2O_2 and soft toothbrush q 4 hr. Once a day, clean teeth with a mixture of H_2O_2 and baking soda to neutralize oral acid and remove plaque.
11. Back care and deep massage with nonastringent lotion to all bony prominences, except areas with urticaria.
12. Institute all safety measures by elevating side rails and pad if client restless or confused, and arrange call light and personal articles within easy reach.
13. Maintain frequent physical and visual contact with client during acute phase stating time of return before leaving.
14. Reorient to time, place, and reason for hospitalization with each contact if client confused or disoriented.
15. Explain condition and progress to client and family with each contact. Assist them to ask questions and express concerns of the present and the future.
16. Obtain Medic-Alert bracelet for client, before discharge.

Change–Interdependent

1. Administer epinephrine 1:1000 strength 0.5 to 0.75 ml by slow IV push or according to protocol, or as prescribed by physician. (Epinephrine is the drug of choice because it decreases mediator release, dilates the bronchioles, and causes vasoconstriction.)
2. Medicate for pain or nausea as prescribed and assess effect in 10 to 20 min.
3. Notify physician if:
    Chemotherapy discontinued due to anaphylaxis stating severity of symptoms exhibited
    Skin test demonstrates wheal of greater than 3 mm
    Hemoglobin greater than 18.0 g/dl males, 16.0 g/dl females
    Hematocrit greater than 52% males, 48% females
    Blood pH less than 7.4
    Po_2 less than 75 torr
    Pco_2 greater than 45 torr
    O_2 saturation less than 90%
    IgE antibody test greater than 1 mg/dl

4. Anticipate physician to prescribe:

Plasma or volume expanders to restore volume and maintain BP

Endotracheal intubation with ventilatory assistance with severe respiratory distress.

Antihistamines to act as competitive antagonist to histamines at receptor site and relieve urticaria

CVP line to monitor venous return with severe hypotension.

Levarterenol (norepinephrine, Levophed) at 4 mg/min to cause vasoconstriction and elevate BP

Aminophylline IV with continued bronchospasm 5 to 6 mg/kg infused over 20 to 30 min initially, followed by 1.0 mg/kg/hr

Note: Corticosteroids, dopamine, and dobutamine are not recommended in the treatment of anaphylaxis.

BIBLIOGRAPHY

Anaphylaxis and the community nurse *Nursing Mirror*, **145**(10), 1977, 41-42.

Arnold, D.J., and Stafford, C.T. Systemic allergic reaction to adriamycin. *Cancer Treat Rep*, **63**, 1979, 150-151 (letter).

Cassmeyer, V. *Medical-surgical nursing—Concepts and clinical practice.* In W.J. Phipps, B.C. Long, and N. Fugate Woods (Eds.), Integrated Mechanisms. St. Louis, C.V. Mosby, 1979, chapt 13, pp. 195-196.

Crossland, J. *Lewis's Pharmacology* (5th ed.) New York: Churchill Livingstone, 1980. pp. 404-411.

Freeman, A.I. Clinical note: Allergic reaction to daunomycin (NSC-82151). *Cancer Chemother Rep*, **54**, 1970, 475-476.

Gluck-Kuyt, I., and Irwin, L.E. Anaphylactic reaction to high-dose methotrexate. *Cancer Treat Rep*, **63**, 1979, 797-798.

Goldberg, N.H., Romolo, J.L., Austin, E.H., Drake, J., and Rosenberg, S. Anaphylactoid type reactions in two patients receiving high dose intravenous methotrexate. *Cancer*, **42**, 1978, 52-55.

Goodman, L.S., and Gillman, A. *The pharmacological basis of therapeutics* (4th ed.). New York: Macmillan, 1970.

Gordon, M. *Manual of nursing diagnosis.* McGraw-Hill, 1982.

Holt, D. Anaphylactic shock: A shock that's easy to see. *Nursing Mirror*, **148**(5), 1979, 31-34.

Karchmer, R.K., and Hansen, V.L. Possible anaphylactic reaction to intravenous Cyclophosphamide: Report of a Case. *JAMA*, 1977, pp. 237-475.

Kreamer, K.M., Anaphylaxis resulting from chemotherapy. *Oncology Nursing Forum*, **8**(4), 1981, 13-16.

Krutchik, A.N., Buzdar, A.U., and Tashima, C.K. Cyclophosphamide-induced urticaria: Occurrence in a patient with no cross-sensitivity to chlorambucil. *Arch Intern Med*, **138**, 1978, 1725-1726.

Lakin, J.D., and Cahill, R.A. Generalized urticaria to cyclophosphamide: Type I hypersensitivity to an immunosuppressive agent. *J Allergy Clin Immunol*, **58**, 1976, 160–171.

Lawrence, B.V., Harvey, H.A., and Lipton, A. Anaphylaxis due to oral melphalan. *Cancer Treatment Reports*, **64**, 1980, 731–732 (letter).

Lind, M. The immunological assessment: A nursing focus. *Heart and Lung*, **19**(4), 1980, 658–661.

Murti, L., and Horsman, L.R. Acute hypersensitivity reaction to cyclophosphamide. *J Pediatr*, **94**, 1979, 844–845.

Ross, W.E., and Chabner, B.A. Allergic reaction to cyclophosphamide in a mechlorethamine-sensitive patient. *Cancer Treat Rep*, **64**, 1977, 495–496.

Souhami, L., Jr., and Field, R. Urticaria following intravenous doxorubicin administration. *JAMA*, **240**, 1978, 1624–1626.

Van Scott, E.J., and Kalmanson, J.D. Complete remissions of mycosis fungoides lymphoma induced by topical nitrogen mustard (HN_2): Control of delayed hypersensitivity to HN_2 by desensitization and by induction of specific immunologic tolerance. *Cancer*, **32**, 1973, 18–30.

Weiss, R.B. Hypersensitivity reaction to cancer chemotherapeutic agents. *Annals of Internal Medicine*, **94**, 1981, 66–72.

Yarbro, J.W., and Bornstein, R.S. *Oncologic emergencies*. New York: Grune and Stratton, 1981.

26. Cell-Mediated Immunity Impairment

DEFINITION AND CAUSATIVE FACTORS

Cell-mediated immunity impairment (CMII) develops in the client with cancer as a result of cytotoxic drugs including azathioprine, cyclophosphamide, cyclosporin A, and steroids, and radiation causing depression of the bone marrow with lymphopenia and leukopenia. With the loss of this important defense mechanism, the immunosuppressed client has an enormous potential for infection and sepsis.

There are 2 types of immunity: nonspecific, which involves the phagocytic action of leukocytes (neutrophils and eosinophils), and specific, which consists of B cell and T cell lymphocytes. B-lymphocytes (Bursa derived) provide humoral immunity producing antigen specific antibodies (immunoglobins) IgG, complement fixation of bacteria, viruses, and some fungi; IgM, complement fixation and agglutination of bacteria; and IgA, IgD, IgE. Cellular immunity of T-lymphocytes (thymus-related) functions to protect against viruses, slow bacteria, fungi in delayed hypersensitivity reactions, in rejection of grafts, and in immunologic surveillance by cytotoxic killer cells, helper T-lymphocytes, and suppressor T cells that prevent the overproduction of antibodies.

The immunologic status of the client is tested by using recall antigens intradermally, candida, mumps virus, purified protein derivative (PPD), streptokinase, streptodornase, and trichophytin. The client is considered anergic if no reaction occurs after 48 hrs. Normally, erythema with induration (raised, reddened wheal) results because of lifetime exposure to these antigens. Dinitrochlorobenzene (DNCB) is used to determine if the body can produce new antibodies because there is no natural immunity to this chemical.

Infection is the leading cause of death in the immunosuppressed client with an incidence of 50 to 79%; 67 to 93% are bacterial, 10 to 25% are fungal, and virus infections constitute about the same incidence as in the general population.

Corresponding cancers include all treated with chemotherapy, specifically lymphomas, Hodgkin, leukemias, and multiple myelomas. Radiation, glucocorticosteroids, malnutrition, and lymph node removal are additional causes.

ASSESSMENT DATA

- Recall antigen test induration less than 10 mm
- DNCB hypersensitivity reaction less than grade 4
- Decreased percentage of T cells and B cells
- Decreased neutrophil (PMN) count—less than 500/mm^3
- Decreased monocyte count—less than 3%
- Decreased lymphocyte count—less than 1,000/mm^3
- Abnormal lymphocyte transformation test
- Increased or normal temperature
- Positive cultures of blood, urine, throat, lesions, vagina
- Productive cough with change in color, amount, consistency of sputum
- Pain, erythema, tenderness of an area

(It may be difficult to diagnose infection in the immunosuppressed client because the normal indications of infection are absent or disguised by the malignancy or therapy. Cultures are the most reliable index as well as changes in data of the nursing assessment.)

NURSING DIAGNOSES

Potential for infection, related to leukopenia and lymphopenia, resulting from bone marrow depression.

RATIONALE

Inability of body to fight infection due to impairment of T cell lymphocytes that are derived from stem cells originating in the bone marrow and formed in the lymphoid tissue of the body.

NURSING INTERVENTIONS

Monitoring–Independent

1. Oral temperature q 2 to 4 hr.
2. Assess client for productive cough with each contact and inspect for changes in color, amount, and consistency of sputum.

3. Auscultate breath sounds in all lung fields q 4 to 8 hr and record onset of adventitious sounds, diminished or absent breath sounds, and pleural friction rub.

4. Assess respiratory rate q 2 to 4 hr and record onset of dyspnea or hyperpnea.

5. Assess skin color, temperature, and moisture q 4 to 8 hr and record presence or changes in skin lesions.

6. Assess LOC q 4 hr and record changes in awareness, orientation, and behavior.

7. BP and heart rate q 4 hr.

8. Accurate I and O, calculate I/O ratio for fluid balance q 8 and 24 hr.

9. Record number, color, and consistency of all stools.

10. Inspect urine q 8 hr for changes in color and odor.

11. Inspect perineum for color and amount of vaginal secretions q 8 hr.

12. Assess oral cavity for white patches, lesions, or odor q 8 hr.

13. Inspect eyes for redness or exudate q 8 hr.

14. Auscultate heart sounds in 4 valvular sites q 8 hr and record onset of extra heart sounds.

15. Auscultate bowel sounds in 4 quadrants q 8 hr and record changes in pitch and frequency.

Monitoring–Interdependent

1. Assess recall antigen skin test in 48 hr by measuring size of induration.
   15 mm: normal
   5 to 10 mm: mild immune depletion
   5 or less: severe immune depletion
   O: anergy
   DNCB: 2 to 5 mm red bumps and graded 0 to 4
   Lymphocyte Transformation Test: normal B, T cell reactions

2. Assess results of laboratory data when available and compare to previous and normal values.
   Lymphocyte Count: 1,000 to 3,000/mm³ (25 to 35%)
   Neutrophil (PMN) Count: 2,500 to 7,000/mm³ (50 to 70%)
   T cell Lymphocytes: 70 to 80%
   B cell Lymphocytes: 5 to 10%
   WBC: 4,500 to 11,500/mm³
   Eosinophils: 4%
   Basophils: 1%
   Monocytes: 5%
   IgG: 800 to 1800 mg/dl
   IgM: 50 to 150 mg/dl

TABLE 26-1. COMMON INFECTIONS IN THE
IMMUNOSUPPRESSED CLIENT WITH CANCER

Organism	Pathogen	Infection
Bacteria	*Pseudomonas aeruginosa*	Septicemia
		Skin infections, wound infections
	Klebsiella	UTI, aspiration pneumonia
	Escherichia coli	UTI, severe diarrhea
	Staphylococcus aureus	Skin infections, pneumonia, meningitis, endocarditis, toxic shock syndrome
Fungus	Candida	Thrush, vaginal infection
	Aspergillus niger	Lung infection
	Cryptococcus neoformans	Cryptococcal pneumonia, meningitis
Virus	Varicella–Zoster	Shingles, fatal in children with cancer
	Herpes simplex	Oropharynx, genital infections, encephalitis
	Cytomegalovirus	Pneumonia, hepatitis, chorioretinitis
Parasite	*Pneumocystis carini*	Interstitial pneumonia
	Toxoplasma gondii	Severe disseminated infection of heart, brain, liver, kidneys

ABGs   pH: 7.35 to 7.45
Po_2: 75 to 100 torr
Pco_2: 35 to 45 torr
HCO_3: 24 to 30 mEq/L
O_2 Saturation: 95 to 100%
CO_2 Content: 24 to 30 mEq/L
BE: ± 2 mEq/L

3. Assess results of cultures and determine possible infectious sites according to Table 26-1.
4. Assess client for appropriate side effects of antibiotic drugs once therapy initiated including superimposed infections.
5. Assess IV site for pain, redness, and swelling q 4 to 8 hr.

Change–Independent

1. Wash hands before and after each client contact for 2 min per hand using antiseptic skin cleansing agent and vigorous friction.
2. Isolate client in private room with bath, away from the utility room or heavy trafficked areas if possible. Leave all equipment in room after cleaning with antiseptic solutions.

3. Screen all visitors and staff for infection and prevent their contact with client if appropriate. (Visitor may use gown and mask and stand at a distance from client.)

4. Maintain bedrest and minimize all activity.

5. Bathe daily, without soap, using commercially prepared bath emollient.

6. Back care and light massage with nonastringent lotion to all bony prominences q 4 hr except skin areas that are abraded or being radiated.

7. Cleanse all skin lesions or breaks with betadine q 4 hr. Deep wounds or incisions should be cleansed and dressed aseptically using prescribed antiseptic.

8. Mouth care using $\frac{1}{2}$ strength H_2O_2 and soft toothbrush q 8 hr. Once a day, clean teeth with a mixture of H_2O_2 and baking soda to neutralize oral acid and remove plaque.

9. Offer bland protein fluids as tolerated q 2 hr.

10. Passive ROME to all major joints q 8 hr.

11. Turn, cough, deep breathe q 2 hr.

12. O_2 at 2 L/min by nasal cannula for onset of dyspnea and elevate HOB to 30 to 60%.

13. Institute all safety measures by elevating side rails and pad if client restless and disoriented, placing bed in low position, and arranging call light and personal articles within easy reach.

14. Explain condition and progress to client and family with each contact. Assist them to ask questions and express concerns of the present and the future.

15. Include family members in plan of care and allow them to participate, if mutually therapeutic.

Change–Interdependent

1. Notify physician if:
   Induration of 10 mm or less with recall antigen skin test
   Lymphocyte count less than 500/mm^3
   Neutrophil count less than 1500/mm^3
   T-lymphocytes less than 70% (unless bone marrow depression therapeutically induced)
   Po$_2$ less than 75 torr
   O_2 saturation less than 90%
   Blood pH less than 7.35
   Onset of adventitious or decreased breath sounds
   Results of positive blood, sputum, vaginal, throat, urine cultures

2. Anticipate physician to prescribe:
   Decrease or change in chemotherapy and/or radiation treatments
   Recall antigen skin tests

DNCB hypersensitivity reaction test

Chest x-rays with alterations in respiratory function or onset of productive sputum

Reverse isolation if client anergic

Eliminating or minimizing invasive procedures or tubes

Laminar air flow room

Antibiotics

Mycostatin mouthwash and swallow

Vaginal antifungal cream or suppository

Blood cultures with temperature elevation greater than 101.0° F

WBC infusions with severe WBC or lymphocyte depletion

3. Consult dietitian for diet consisting of cooked foods only.

BIBLIOGRAPHY

Axnick, K.J. Infection control considerations in the care of the immunosuppressed patient. *Critical Care Quarterly*, 3(12), 1980, 79–88.

Brody, N. Laboratory tests to evaluate cell-mediated immunity. *Cutis*, **28**, 1981, 575–577.

Corbett, J.V. *Laboratory tests in nursing practice*. Norwalk, Connecticut: Appleton-Century-Crofts, 1982.

Donoghue, M., Nunnally, C., and Yasko, J.M. *Nutritional aspects of cancer care*. Virginia: Reston, 1982.

Gordon, M. *Manual of Nursing Diagnosis*. New York: McGraw-Hill, 1982.

Groenwald, S.L. Physiology of the immune system. *Heart and Lung*, **9**(4), 1980, 645–650.

Kee, J.L. *Laboratory and diagnostic tests with nursing implications*. Norwalk, Connecticut: Appleton-Century-Crofts, 1983.

Lind, M. The immunologic assessment: A nursing focus. *Heart and Lung*, **9**(4), 1980, 658–661.

Rana, A.N., and Luskin, A. Immunosuppression, autoimmunity, and hypersensitivity. *Heart and Lung*, **9**(4), 1980, 651–657.

Thomas, L. On immunosurveillance in human cancer. *The Yale Journal of Biology and Medicine*, **55**, 1982, 329–333.

27. Graft-Versus-Host Disease

DEFINITION AND CAUSATIVE FACTORS

Graft-versus-host disease (GVHD) develops in the client with leukemia who has received a bone marrow transplant (BMT) in which the donor cells attack and kill the host cells. It is characterized as acute or chronic, involves skin, GI tract, liver, and bone marrow, and is graded from I to IV according to its severity (Tables 27-1 and 27-2). GVHD is initiated by the donor T cells, cell-mediated lymphocytes that function in delayed sensitivity reactions, tumor immunity, and graft rejection by multiplying to attack antigens so that the reticuloendothelial system can destroy them. The donor T cells, contained in BMT, proliferate and target various normal cells in the immunosuppressed host who is immunologically incompetent to fight these invaders. Acute GVHD occurs in clients within 7 to 14 days following BMT, and skin manifestations are the first symptoms. Chronic GVHD has a 10% incidence and may develop following the acute phase or from 2 to 12 months after transplantation. Infection and hemorrhage are the most serious complications.

Prior to BMT, the client usually has total body radiation and intravenous Methotrexate or cyclosporin A to completely suppress all bone marrow activity. Tissue typing is determined for donor HL-A (human lymphocyte antigen) compatibility. Only identical twins are completely HL-A compatible, and there is a current emphasis on autologous bone transplants obtained when the client is in remission which would eliminate the possibility of GVHD. Clients who are presensitized to blood products because of multiple transfusions have a greater risk; therefore, all blood and blood products are irradiated to cease T cell growth. Despite these measures, GVHD has a 50 to 70% incidence with bone marrow transplantation, and the long-term effects include dermal sclerosis, inelasticity, contractures, stomatitis, dry eye syndrome, and corneal opacification.

Corresponding cancer includes leukemia. Severe radiation exposure, aplastic anemia, congenital immunodeficiency diseases, presensitization with previous blood transfusions, and histoincompatibility are additional causes.

TABLE 27-1. PROPOSED CLINICAL STAGE OF GRAFT-VERSUS-HOST DISEASE ACCORDING TO ORGAN SYSTEM

+	Maculopapular rash <25% body surface	Bilirubin 2–3 mg/100 ml	>500 ml diarrhea/day
++	Maculopapular rash 25–50% body surface	Bilirubin 3–6 mg/100 ml	>1000 ml diarrhea/day
+++	Generalized erythroderma	Bilirubin 6–15 mg/100 ml	>1500 ml diarrhea/day
++++	Generalized erythroderma with bullous formation and desquamation	Billirubin >15 mg/100 ml	Severe abdominal pain, with or without ileus

(Source: from Thomas, E.D. Bone marrow transplantation. *New England Journal of Medicine*, **292**, 1975, 896, with permission).

ASSESSMENT DATA

- Skin
  Stage I   Pruritic, faint red, maculopapular eruptions on face, forehead, palms and soles.

  Stage II   Rash extends to trunk with peeling and turns to a deep red color.

  Stage III Generalized erythroderma.

  Stage IV   Blistering and sloughing turning bronze in color with healing.

  Chronic   From erythroderma to sclerosis, hypo- or hyperpigmentation, inelasticity; contractures of wrist, fingers, knees, insteps; thickened nails, damage to the lacrimal ducts, salivary glands and sweat glands resulting in stomatitis, conjunctivitis, and corneal opacification.

TABLE 27-2. CLINICAL GRADING OF SEVERITY OF GRAFT-VERSUS-HOST DISEASE

Grade	Degree of Organ Involvement
I	+ to ++ skin rash; no gut involvement; no liver involvement; no decrease in clinical performance
II	+ to +++ skin rash; + gut involvement or + liver involvement (or both); mild decrease in clinical performance
III	++ to +++ skin rash; ++ to +++ gut involvement or ++ to ++++ liver involvement (or both); marked decrease in clinical performance
IV	Similar to grade III with ++ to ++++ organ involvement and extreme decrease in clinical performance

(Source: from Thomas, E.D. Bone marrow transplantation. *New England Journal of Medicine*, **292**, 1975, 896, with permission.)

- GI tract
    Green, watery, guaiac positive stools as severe as 6 to 7 L/day
    Anorexia
    Nausea, vomiting
    Abdominal pain
    Malabsorption
    Paralytic ileus
    Ascites
- Liver
    Increased SGOT, bilirubin, alkaline phosphatase, and LDH
    Fatigue
    Malaise
    Jaundice
    Bilirubinuria
    Fever
    Hepatomegaly
    Hemorrhage
    Liver biopsy—lymphocyte infiltration with hepatocellular and bile
        duct necrosis
- Bone marrow
    Pancytopenia
    Fatigue
    Pallor
    Infection
- Vaginal adhesions, stenosis, and inflammation

NURSING DIAGNOSES	RATIONALE
Impaired skin integrity, related to rash, blistering, sloughing, resulting from donor T-lymphocyte reaction to the epidermal and dermal cells of the host.	*Deposits of IgM antibodies at the dermal–epidermal junction destroy skin cells.*

Associated Nursing Diagnoses

1. Nutritional deficit, related to degeneration of the gastric mucosal cells caused by a donor T-lymphocyte reaction, resulting in severe diarrhea, nausea, and vomiting.

Degeneration of the mucosa and mucosal glands.

2. Potential for infection, related to pancytopenia, resulting from a donor T-lymphocyte reaction causing bone marrow depression.

Mild to severe suppression of WBC, RBC, and platelets.

3. Body image disturbance, related to skin sloughing, scarring, and alterations in pigmentation, resulting from a donor T-lymphocyte reaction to the skin cells of the host.

Physical change alters perception, feelings, and attitude. Psychologic investment in our body appearance is derived from physical, environmental, and cultural factors.

4. Sensory deficit, sight, related to corneal opacification and dry eye syndrome occurring in chronic GVHD, resulting from damage to the lacrimal ducts.

Pre-BMT treatment as well as T-lymphocyte reactions posttransplant cause ocular problems.

NURSING INTERVENTIONS

Monitoring–Independent

1. Assess skin for maculopapular rash q 2 hr after bone marrow transplant and describe location and stage.

    Stage I   Faint red maculopapular rash on face, forehead, palms, and soles of feet
    Stage II   Rash extends to trunk turning deep red with peeling
    Stage III   Generalized erythroderma
    Stage IV   Sloughing areas turn bronze in color with healing

2. Assess degree of itching and presence of scleral jaundice with each client contact.

3. Assess client with skin changes on admission with chronic GVHD and describe.

    Location and degree of contractures
    Presence of stomatitis
    Presence of conjunctivitis and/or drug eye syndrome
    Degree of sight impairment with corneal opacification
    Location and degree of skin scarring
    Limitation in ADLs resulting from contractures, sight impairment, and scarring
    Feelings and attitude toward changes in body image

4. Assess all body surfaces for infected areas as evidenced by heat, pain, redness, swelling, and exudate q 8 hr.

5. Assess eye surfaces for dryness or clouding of the cornea q 8 hr.
6. Temperature q 4 hr.
7. Measure and describe all diarrheal stools.
8. Assess client for nausea with each contact and anorexia at mealtime.
9. Auscultate bowel sounds in 4 quadrants q 8 hr and record location of changes in pitch and frequency.
10. Palpate abdomen q 4 to 8 hr for distention, rigidity, general, and rebound tenderness.
11. Hemocult all emesis, stools, and inspect urine for hematuria.
12. BP, heart rate, and respirations q 2 to 4 hr.
13. Assess client for objective and subjective indications of fatigue, weakness, or malaise with each contact.
14. Accurate I and O, calculate I/O ratio for fluid balance q 8 and 24 hr.
15. Weigh q AM before breakfast and compare to previous measurements.
16. Assess LOC q 8 hr and record changes in awareness, orientation, and behavior.
17. Assess IV or TPN site for redness, pain, or swelling q 4 to 8 hr.
18. Assess for vaginitis q week following BMT.

Monitoring–Interdependent

1. Assess results of laboratory data when available and compare to previous and normal values.

    CBC   Hemoglobin: 13.0 to 18.0 g/dl males
                        12.0 to 16.0 g/dl females
            Hematocrit: 45 to 52% males
                    37 to 48% females
            RBC: 4.6 to 6.2 × 10^6/mm^3 males
                4.2 to 5.4 × 10^6/mm^3 females
            MCHC: 32 to 36%
            MCH: 27 to 32 pg
            MCV: 80 to 94 cu microns
            Platelets: 130,000 to 370,000 mm^3
            WBC: 4,500 to 11,500/mm^3
  Differential   Bands: 3 to 5%
                    Neutrophils: 51 to 67%
                    Eosinophils: 1 to 4%
                    Basophils: 0 to 1%
                    Lymphocytes: 25 to 33%
                    Monocytes: 2 to 6%

Serum Sodium: 135 to 145 mEq/L
Serum Potassium: 3.5 to 5.0 mEq/L
Serum Chloride: 100 to 106 mEq/L
Serum Calcium: 8.5 to 10.5 mg/dl
Serum Protein: 6.0 to 8.4 g/dl
Serum Bilirubin: total 1.0 mg/dl
                  indirect: 0.6 mg/dl
Alkaline phosphatase: 13 to 39 IU
SGOT: 60 to 120 U/ml
LDH: 10 to 40 U/ml

Change–Independent

1. Maintain bedrest with limited activity with onset of infection, anemia, or extreme fatigue and weakness.
2. Lubricate skin with half mineral oil and half A & D ointment twice a day.
3. Apply 2 gtts artificial tears solution to both eyes q 2 to 4 hr.
4. Apply sterile vaseline gauze followed by dry sterile dressing to all open areas.
5. Perirectal care after all diarrheal stools and apply protective agent.
6. Apply ice collar to neck with indications of nausea or vomiting.
7. Mouth care q 2 hr, after meals and after all vomiting episodes using $\frac{1}{2}$ strength H_2O_2 and soft tooth brush. Once a day, clean teeth with a mixture of H_2O_2 and baking soda to neutralize oral acid and remove plaque.
8. Offer bland protein fluids and nonirritating juices q 2 hr as tolerated.
9. Bathe daily without soap using betadine solution or other prescribed antiseptic solution.
10. Turn, cough, deep breathe q 2 hr while on bedrest.
11. Passive ROME to all major joints as tolerated q 4 hr.
12. O_2 at 2 L/min by nasal cannula with SOB induced by a low hemoglobin.
13. Back care q 4 hr using nonastringent lotion to all unaffected bony areas.
14. Assist client to perform ADLs and maintain judicious independence and control over self and environment within physical limitations.
15. File fingernails to shortest length and gently brush clean qd.
16. Apply mittens to prevent scratching, if necessary.
17. Institute all safety measures with onset of weakness and fatigue by elevating side rails, placing bed in low position, and arranging call light and personal articles within easy reach.
18. Prevent visitors and staff with infections from visiting client (or use protocol for laminar air flow room).

19. Explain condition and progress to client and family with each contact. Assist them to ask questions and express concerns of the present and the future.

Change–Interdependent

1. Notify physician if:
   Rash appears after bone marrow transplant
   Persistent vomiting or diarrhea occurs
   Temperature elevates to 101.0° F or more
   Bowel sounds become high pitched and hyperactive or hypoactive/absent
   SGOT greater than 120 U/ml
   LDH greater than 40 U/ml
   Hemoglobin less than 10 g/dl
   Hematocrit less than 30%
   Serum sodium less than 135 mEq/L or greater than 145 mEq/L
   Serum potassium less than 3.5 mEq/L
   Serum calcium less than 8.5 mg/dl
   Melena, hematemesis, or hematuria occurs
   Platelets less than 130,000 mm³
   WBC greater than 12,000/mm³
   Vaginitis appears after bone marrow transplant

2. Anticipate physician to prescribe:
   Reverse isolation or laminar air flow room to prevent infection
   Corticosteroids to prevent proliferation of T cells
   IV antithymocyte globulin to destroy donor lymphocytes but is toxic to RBC and platelets. Benedryl and Solu-medrol may be needed to counteract hypersensitivity
   WBC transfusions to prevent infection
   Antibiotics
   Parenteral antiemetics
   Antacids to neutralize gastric acids
   IV Tagamet to prevent ulcer formation
   TPN if severe vomiting occurs for 3 days or more duration
   NG tube if paralytic ileus suspected
   Imuran (azathioprine) for chronic GVHD to suppress T cell reactions
   Phase I clinical trial upon consent of client—clinical research associated with chemotherapy drug investigation whose aim is to establish a maximal tolerated dose and then arrive at an optimal dose for phase II trials.
   Phase II clinical trial upon request of client—clinical research whose purpose is to demonstrate whether newly developed compounds have a useful clinical effect in certain tumors.

BIBLIOGRAPHY

Brown, M.H., and Kiss, M.E. Standards of care for the patient with graft-versus-host disease post-bone marrow transplant. *Cancer Nursing*, 4(3), 1981, 191–198.

Corbett, J.V. *Laboratory tests in nursing practice*. Norwalk, Connecticut: Appleton-Century-Crofts, 1982.

Corson, S.L., et al. Gynecologic manifestations of chronic graft-versus-host disease. *Obstetrics and Gynecology*, 60(4), 1982, 488–492.

DiJulio, J.E., and Bedigian, J.S. Hybridoma monoclonal antibody treatment of T cell lymphomas: Clinical experience and nursing management. *Oncology Nursing Forum*, 10(2), 1983, 22–27.

Gordon, M. *Manual of nursing diagnosis*. New York: McGraw-Hill, 1982.

Jack, M., and Hicks, J. Ocular complications in high-dose chemoradiotherapy and marrow transplantation. *Annals of Ophthalmology*, 13, 1981, 709–711.

Nursing Grand Rounds. Going the distance with the patient who's a real fighter. *Nursing 83*, 1983, pp 70–75.

Owen, H., Klove, C., and Cotanch, P.H. Bone marrow harvesting and high-dose BCNU therapy: Nursing implications. *Cancer Nursing*, 4(3), 1981, 199–205.

Rice, L., Schottstaedt, M., Udden, M., and Jackson, D. Transplantation of bone marrow: Graft-vs.-host disease. *Heart and Lung*, 10(5), 1981, 897–900.

Roy, C., Ghayur, T., Kongshavn, P.A.L., and Lapp, W.S. Natural killer activity by spleen, lymph node, and thymus cells during the graft-versus-host reaction. *Transplantation*, 34(3), 1982, 144–146.

Serota, F.T., Rosenberg, H.K., Rosen, J., Koch, P.A., and August, C.S. Delayed onset of gastrointestinal disease in the recipients of bone marrow transplantation—A variant graft-versus-host reaction. *Transplantation*, 34(1), 1982, 60–64.

Tsoi, M.S. Immunological mechanisms of graft-versus-host disease in man. *Transplantation*, 33(5), 1982, 459–464.

PART V
MOBILITY

28. Pathologic Fractures

DEFINITION AND CAUSATIVE FACTORS

Pathologic fracture occurs with bone metastasis from high risk corresponding cancers. There is a 33% incidence of bone metastasis in all clients with cancer, and 8% will develop fractures. There is no difference in survival rates between single or multiple pathologic fractures. The most susceptible bones are those with greatest bone marrow activity and blood flow which include vertebrae, pelvis, ribs, proximal long bones, skull, and sternum. Bone metastasis develops most commonly by tumor emboli through the venous circulation although direct invasion is also possible. The first indication of bone involvement is pain, which increases with activity, and is not relieved with rest. Pain often occurs before radiologic visualization.

Spinal metastasis occurs from primaries of the breast, lung, prostate, lymphoma, and plasma cell myeloma involving T-9 to L-4. Cervical metastasis is less common and is indicated by loss of neck rotation, paresthesia, weakness, and incontinuence. Metastasis to the ribs and sternum is caused by cancer of the breast, lung, thyroid, kidney, and lymphoma which produces pain with respirations. Malignant effusion, erosion into the pleura, and fat emboli are hazardous sequelae. The femur and humerus are the most common sites of long bone metastasis, and this is usually a result of sarcomas. X-ray changes will not develop until 30 to 60% of the bone has been destroyed, although a bone scan will demonstrate metastasis somewhat earlier.

Other corresponding cancers include ovary, colorectal, pancreas, and stomach. Uremia, vitamin D deficiency, previous bone radiation, hypocalcemia, and hypophosphatemia are additional causes.

ASSESSMENT DATA

- History of known malignancy
- Pain in back, neck, extremities
- Crepitus in involved area

- Edema of surrounding tissue
- Increased serum alkaline phosphatase
- Increased serum acid phosphatase fractionation (for prostatic cancers)
- X-ray or bone scan indication
- Increased serum calcium and phosphorus with demineralization of bone
- Increased WBC and erythrocyte sedimentation rate (Ewing sarcoma)

NURSING DIAGNOSES	RATIONALE
Impaired physical mobility, level I, related to destruction of the vertebrae, pelvis, or long bones, resulting in loss of function necessary for mobility because of pathologic fracture.	*Bone destruction decreases actual bone strength and movement within the environment.*

Associated Nursing Diagnoses

1. Alteration in comfort, related to bone pain, resulting from bone metastasis, demineralization, and fracture.	Pain results from the fracture site and the surrounding edematous tissue.
2. Ineffective breathing patterns, related to demineralization and possible fracture of ribs and sternum, which interferes with chest expansion necessary for respiration, resulting in hypoventilation.	The principal danger of fractured ribs is pleural puncture causing pneumothorax. Pain on inspiration limits the respiratory excursion.
3. Potential alteration in bowel elimination, related to constipation, resulting from prolonged bedrest following a pathologic fracture.	Intestinal motility is decreased during prolonged bedrest.

NURSING INTERVENTIONS

Monitoring–Independent

1. Assess alignment of bones of the vertebrae, arms, legs, and pelvis and ability to move on command q 8 hr with onset of bone pain.

2. Palpate bones of vertebrae, arms, legs, and pelvis for tenderness and crepitus with onset of bone pain q 8 hr.

3. Assess for pain (with and without weight bearing) in neck, back, chest, arms, and legs with each contact and describe:
   Location
   Intensity at rest and with movement
   Radiation
   Duration
   Presence of crepitus in painful area

4. Assess for ease and depth of inspiration, tracheal position, and symmetry of chest movement with each client contact with complaints of chest pain on inspiration and expiration and record onset of dyspnea, paradoxical chest movement, and tracheal shift.

5. Auscultate breath sounds in all lung fields q 8 hr and record onset of adventitious sounds.

6. Assess for cough and record color and consistency of sputum.

7. Assess LOC q 4 to 8 hr and record changes in awareness, orientation, and behavior.

8. Assess skin color, temperature, moisture, and discolorations q 8 hr (petechiae on chest and shoulders are indications of fat emboli).

9. Oral temperature q 4 hr.

10. Assess for Homan sign in unaffected lower extremity with prolonged bedrest q 8 hr.

11. BP, heart rate, and respirations q 4 hr.

12. Auscultate heart sounds in 4 valvular sites q 8 hr and record onset of extra heart sounds.

13. Accurate I and O and calculate I/O ratio for fluid balance q 8 and 24 hr.

14. Auscultate bowel sounds in 4 quadrants q 8 hr and record pitch and frequency of sound.

15. Assess bowel function by noting date of last bowel movement qd.

Monitoring–Interdependent

1. Assess results of laboratory data when available and compare to previous and normal values.
   Serum Alkaline Phosphatase: 13 to 39 IU
   Serum Calcium: 8.5 to 10.5 mg/dl
   Serum Phosphorus: 3.0 to 4.5 mg/dl
   Serum Uric Acid: 3.0 to 7.0 mg/dl
   ABGs   pH: 7.35 to 7.45
             Po_2: 75 to 100 torr

Pco_2: 35 to 45 torr
HCO_3: 24 to 30 mEq/L
CO_2 Content: 24 to 30 mEq/L
BE: $\pm$ 2 mEq/L
O_2 Saturation: 95 to 100%
WBC: 4,500 to 11,500/mm^3
Erythrocyte Sedimentation Rate (ESR)
(Cutler Method): Male 0 to 8 mm/hr
                                Female 0 to 10 mm/hr
Under 50 years old: Male 0 to 15 mm/hr
(Westergren Method): Female 0 to 20 mm/hr
Over 50 years old: Male 0 to 20 mm/hr
(Westergren Method): Female 0 to 30 mm/hr

Drugs that influence an increased sedimentation rate (associated with Ewing sarcoma) include dextran, Aldomet, Sansert, Pronestyl, theophylline, and oral contraceptives.

2. Assess results of x-rays or bone scan.
3. With application of splint or brace to immobilize fracture.
   Remove splint or brace q 8 hr and assess skin for abrasions, reddened areas, or blisters.
   Assess all areas under splint or brace for pain, pressure sensations, or paresthesias.
   Assess areas distal to splint or brace for pulses, movement, tissue perfusion, edema, color, and temperature of skin.
4. With application of a cast to immobilize fracture:
   Assess exposed skin around cast and cast edges q 1 hr until dry, then q 8 hr.
   Assess neurovascular integrity of area distal to cast:
   Pulse
   Capillary refill by blanching test
   Motor function on command
   Color, temperature, edema of skin
   Tactile perception
   Muscle strength
   Assess cast for drainage, hot spots, or pain with each client contact.
5. With open reduction and internal fixation of metastasized bone to prevent or immobilize fractures:
   Assess incision q 4 to 8 hr for redness, swelling, presence of exudate, and pain.
   Assess positioning of limb as prescribed by physician with each client contact.
   Assess neurovascular integrity q 4 to 8 hr.

Change–Independent

1. Maintain bedrest with onset of bone pain.
2. O_2 at 2 L/min by nasal cannula with onset of dyspnea.
3. Position unaffected bones for maximum alignment and protect with pillows or other padding devices.
4. Institute all safety measures by elevating side rails, padding side rails if client restless or confused, and placing call light and personal articles within reach.
5. Position affected area of fracture for maximum alignment and therapeutic immobilization and minimal pain.
6. Turn q 2 hr using log roll technique if spine is involved.
7. Cough and deep breathe 3 to 5 times q 2 hr.
8. Back care and deep massage to all bony areas with lotion q 4 hr except areas of radiation and record signs of tissue ischemia and trauma.
9. Passive ROME to all unaffected limb joints q 4 hr and record degree of discomfort.
10. Mouth care with soft toothbrush using appropriate oral antiseptic after meals and at bedtime. Once a day, cleanse teeth with a mixture of H_2O_2 and baking soda to neutralize oral acid and remove plaque.
11. Offer fluids to 200 ml q 1 hr unless contraindicated alternating between fat free milk and juice.
12. Teach client active ROME if appropriate.
    Isotonic exercise techniques with trapeze and footboard q 2 hr
    Isometric exercise techniques of contracting and relaxing muscle groups q alternate 2 hr
    Ambulation with assistance for weightbearing or as prescribed by physician
13. Assist client to perform ADLs and maintain judicious independence and control over self and environment within physical limitations.
14. Explain condition and progress to client and family with each contact. Assist them to ask questions and express concerns of the present and future.
15. Include family members in plan of care and allow them to participate, if mutually beneficial.

Change–Interdependent

1. Medicate appropriately for pain as prescribed and assess effect in 10 to 20 min.

2. Notify physician if:
    Bone pain, crepitus, or malalignment develops at site or limb other than present fracture
    Dyspnea or respiratory distress occurs with complaints of chest pain
    Temperature elevates greater than 101.0° F
    WBC greater than 12,000/mm^3
    Petechia develops over shoulders and trunk
    No bowel movement for 4 or more days or client discomfort from lack of defecation
    Positive Homan sign occurs
    Serum calcium levels less than 8.0 mg/dl
    Serum phosphorus levels less than 3.0 mg/dl
    Area distal to cast has pain, edema, numbness, absence of pulse, and decreased movement at will; pale, cool, or cyanotic skin or paresthesia
    Casted area develops hot spot, drainage (serosanguinous or purulent), or odor (musty or foul)
    Erythrocyte sedimentation rate increased.
3. Consult with physician to prescribe diet high in fiber, protein, and calcium if appropriate.
4. Consult with dietitian about assessing client's food preferences and providing 6 small meals per day.
5. Consult with physical therapist (if prescribed) about specific exercise routines appropriate to client's condition and reinforce physical therapist's teaching.
6. Consult with respiratory therapist (if prescribed) for possible benefits of incentive spirometry, IPPB, and other methods of maximizing pulmonary function and preventing complications depending on condition of client.
7. Anticipate physician to prescribe:
    Stabilization device—splint, cast, brace
    Surgical intervention (prophylactic) with open reduction internal fixation (ORIF) and bone cement. Survival is greater with prophylactic ORIF prior to occurrence of fracture with bone metastasis than ORIF after the fracture occurs.
    Radiation to fracture
    Chemotherapy
    Pain medication
    Stool softeners
    ABGs with pulmonary complications or pathologic rib fractures
    Measures to correct hypocalcemia
    Immunoelectrophoresis and serum electrophoresis to detect abnormal proteins in plasm and/or urine for plasma cell myeloma

Laminography
Angiogram
Bone scan
Needle biopsy
TED hose to unaffected leg

BIBLIOGRAPHY

Burns, N. *Nursing and cancer.* Philadelphia: W.B. Saunders, 1982.

Corbett, J.V. *Laboratory tests in nursing practice.* Norwalk, Connecticut: Appleton-Century-Crofts, 1982.

del Regato, J.A., and Spjut, H.L. *Cancer—Diagnosis, treatment, and prognosis* (5th ed.). St. Louis: C.V. Mosby, 1977.

Fidler, M. Incidence of fracture through metastases in long bones. *Acta Orthop. Scand.,* **52,** 1981, 623–627.

Gordon, M. *Manual of nursing diagnosis.* New York: McGraw-Hill, 1982.

Guthrie, H.A. *Introductory nutrition* (4th ed.). St. Louis: C.V. Mosby, 1979.

Hurd, D.D., Thompson, R.C., and Kennedy, B.J. Management of pathologic fractures. In J. Yarbro and R. Bornstein (Eds.), *Oncologic emergencies.* New York: Grune and Stratton, 1981.

Kee, J.L. *Laboratory and diagnostic tests with nursing implications.* Norwalk, Connecticut: Appleton-Century-Crofts, 1983.

Luckman, J., and Sorensen, K.C. *Medical–surgical nursing—A psychophysiologic approach* (2nd ed.). Philadelphia: W.B. Saunders, 1980.

29. Intracerebral Metastasis

DEFINITION AND CAUSATIVE FACTORS

Malignant mestastasis to the brain has a 12 to 24% incidence with invasion primarily to the cerebrum; the cerebellum and brain stem are less frequently involved. The onset of symptoms can be insidious or rapid, and parenchymal brain invasion can develop into a life-threatening situation when compression, edema, or obstruction of cerebral spinal fluid (CSF) cause upward herniation through the tentorial notch or downward herniation through the foramen magnum. Tumor cells from the primary site travel through the arterial circulation and cross the blood–brain barrier causing either single (47%) or multiple (53%) metastasis. Lung cancer and melanoma usually result in multiple metastasis, and breast and renal cancer result in single metastasis. Most chemotherapeutic agents do not cross the blood–brain barrier so that although systemic drugs are controlling the primary tumor, migratory malignant cells can be proliferating in cerebral tissue. The manifestations of intracerebral metastasis depend on the area of the brain involved and are classified as general or focal symptoms. General symptoms are caused by increased intracranial pressure (ICP) with obstruction of CSF flow, and focal symptoms are caused by local compression and destruction of tissue by the malignant mass and edema.

Corresponding cancers include lung, breast, melanoma, testicular, prostate, thyroid, gastric, renal, neuroblastoma, and leukemia.

ASSESSMENT DATA

I. General (increased ICP)
   Change in LOC—restlessness, irritability, memory loss, somnolence, loss of concentration are the first indications of increased ICP which progress eventually to coma (Table 29-1).

TABLE 29-1. CHANGES THAT OCCUR AS THE LEVEL OF CONSCIOUSNESS DECREASES.

Normal consciousness ↓	1. Spontaneous (voluntary) speech at a normal rate. Normal voluntary and reflex somatic motor activity. Eyes open; normal oculomotor activity.
Lethargy	2. Spontaneous sentences, spoken slowly. Decreased speed of voluntary motor activity. Eyes open; decreased oculomotor activity.
	3. Spontaneous words, spoken infrequently. Decreased speed and coordination of voluntary motor activity. Eyes open or closed; decreased oculomotor activity.
Stupor	4. Vocalization only to stimuli that cause pain. Greatly decreased spontaneous motor activity. Eyes generally closed; some spontaneous eye movements.
	5. No vocalization. Appropriate defensive movements, generally flexor, to stimuli that cause pain. Eyes generally closed.
	6. No vocalization. Mass movements to stimuli that cause pain. Eyes closed; decreased spontaneous conjugate eye movements.
Coma	7. No vocalization. Decerebrate posturing to stimuli that cause pain, or no response. Eyes closed; absent spontaneous eye movements.

(Source: from Conway-Rutkowski, B.L. (Ed.). *Carini and Owen's neurological and neurosurgical nursing* (8th ed.). St. Louis: C.V. Mosby, 1982, with permission.)

Headache—worse after awakening or after performing Valsalva maneuver (bending, straining, coughing, sneezing), and are usually bifrontal or bioccipital.

Vomiting—does not have to be projectile and occurs more frequently with cerebellum and brain stem metastasis.

Seizures—occur frequently in multiple intercranial lesions and can be both generalized or focal. (Table 29-2)

Pupillary changes—compression by herniation into the tentorial notch for the third cranial nerve results in ipsilateral pupil dilatation. (For other cranial nerve involvement, see Table 29-2.)

Increasing systolic blood pressure with widening pulse pressure—usually a later sign of increased ICP, accompanied by bradycardia and changes in respiratory pattern. Cheyne–Stokes, tachypnea, or slow shallow respirations are some examples of abnormal patterns.

Papilledema—usually late sign caused by obstruction of venous drainage of optic nerve and retina.

TABLE 29-2. CRANIAL NERVE ASSESSMENT IN INCREASED INTRACRANIAL PRESSURE.

Nerve	Function	Clinical Manifestations
I. Olefactory	Smell	↓ or change in smell
II. Optic	Vision	↓ vision Visual field defect Accident proneness Papilledema
III. Oculomotor IV. Trochlear VI. Abducens	Regular eye movements Pupillary reactions and eyelid movement	Diplopia Abnormal EOMs Nystagmus Unequal or dilated pupil(s) Ptosis
V. Trigeminal	Mastication Facial sensation	Difficulty chewing ↓ or change in facial sensation ↓ or absent corneal reflex

VII. Facial	Facial expression
	Taste—anterior
	  2/3 tongue
	Saliva and tear gland
	  secretion
		Facial weakness/paralysis
		↓ taste
		
		↑ or ↓ saliva and/or tears

VIII. Auditory (vestibulococlear)	Hearing Equilibrium	↓ or loss of hearing Tinnitus Nystagmus Vertigo

IX. Glossopharyn-
  geal
	Swallowing
	Taste—posterior
	  1/3 tongue
		Dysphagia
		↓ taste

X. Vagus	Voice	Hoarseness Dysphagia Deviation of uvula

XI. Spinal
  accessory
	Head, neck and
	  shoulder movement
		Neck and/or shoulder weakness

XII. Hypoglossal	Movement of tongue	Fasciculations, asymmetry, deviations or atrophy of tongue

(Source: from Ryan, L.S., 1981, with permission.)

II. Focal–Cerebral (compression and edema)

Aphasia if left hemisphere involved and dominant (95% of population have dominant left hemispheres).

Weakness, hemiparesis, convulsions wth precentral area (frontal lobe) involvement.

Vision changes in acuity with occipital area involvement.

Affect changes with frontal lobe involvement.

Unable to recognize familiar objects, people, places, and unable to perform routine ADLs with right hemisphere or nondominant involvement.

Focal–Cerebellar

Muscle uncoordination

Ataxia

CT scan, EEG, radionuclide brain scan, and angiography indicative of cerebral metastasis.

A lumbar puncture is contraindicated with increased ICP because it could precipitate herniation.

NURSING DIAGNOSES

Alteration in tissue perfusion related to tumor metastasis causing a decrease in LOC and behavioral charges resulting from increased ICP.

Associated Nursing Diagnoses

1. Alteration in comfort level, acute pain, related to headache, resulting from increased ICP.

2. Sensory deficit related to stereognosis, visual changes, and inappropriate affect resulting from nerve compression from increased ICP.

3. Alteration in mobility, decreased, related to lack of muscle coordination and ataxia resulting from compression of motor tracts.

RATIONALE

The brain, cerebral spinal fluid and blood volume are confined to a nonexpandable space. Any increase in these three cranial volumes causes increased ICP and neurologic deficits.

Traction on the dura from the expanding tumor mass causes acute pain.

Pressure pushes on midbrain causing visual alterations. Expanding tumor mass in frontal lobe causes change in affect.

Cerebellar dysfunction precipitates alterations in mobility.

NURSING INTERVENTIONS

Monitoring–Independent

1. Assess LOC with each client contact and record onset of changes in orientation, awareness, and behavior describing even subtle behavior alterations.
2. Record all seizure activity with each contact and describe according to behavior (Table 29-3).
3. Assess client for headache after awakening and with each contact.
4. Assess client for nausea with each contact and record number of emesis episodes.
5. Inspect bilateral pupil responses q 2 hr for
   Direct light reflex
   Consensual light reflex
   Accommodation—convergence and constriction
   Sluggish or brisk reaction
   Size and equality

TABLE 29-3. SEIZURE ACTIVITY CHART

Classification	Name	Area	Behavior
Partial–simple	Focal motor (Jacksonian March)	Cerebral cortex	Loss of consciousness only if bilateral. Tonic, contraction of sets of muscles, convulsions and clonic contraction, alternating sets of muscles, in extremity or face spreading throughout body.
	Adversive	Frontal area	No loss of consciousness. Head and eyes move away from side of lesion.
	Tonic postural	Cortex	No loss of consciousness. Head turns to one side with tonic extension of extremity.
	Focal sensory	Occipital or parietal	No loss of consciousness. Flashing lights, tingling, numbness, tonic–clonic movements, and odd posturing.
Generalized	Grand-mal, tonic–clonic, major motor.	Cortex Spinal cord	Loss of consciousness, aura, eyes rollup, muscle spasms, and rigidity followed by general twitching and sleep.

(Source: adapted from Conway-Rutkowski B.L. (Ed.). *Carini and Owen's Neurological and neurosurgical nursing* (8th ed.). St. Louis: C. V. Mosby, 1982, with permission.)

6. Assess visual acuity by asking client to read aloud a short printed passage q 8 hr and record subjective complaints of blurred or double vision.

7. Assess hearing acuity by asking client to perform simple commands in varying voice volumes q 8 hr and record changes.

8. Test client's ability to move purposefully by moving extremities on commmand and appropriately responding to painful stimuli q 8 hr.

9. Test muscle strength in extremities by firmness of hand grip and ability to push nurse's hand away with foot using counterforce q 8 hr.

10. BP, heart rate and respiratory rate and pattern q 1 hr with indications of increase ICP and record pulse pressure and onset of changes in heart and respiratory rate.

11. Accurate I and O, calculate I/O ratio for fluid balance q 8 and 24 hr.

12. Urine specific gravity q 8 hr.

13. Record onset of difficult or absent speech.

14. Assess client for activity tolerance and unsteady gait with each contact and record ataxia, subjective indications of weakness and fatigue.

15. Temperature q 4 hr.

Monitoring–Interdependent

1. Monitor intracranial pressure q 2 hr or as prescribed if applicable and compare to previous and normal values.
     4 to 15 torr
     50 to 200 mm H_2O

2. Note x-ray and EEG results indicative of intracerebral metastasis.

3. Assess ICP monitoring site of ventriculostomy reservoir or subarachnoid screw for redness, pain, and swelling q 8 hr.

Change–Independent

1. Maintain bedrest and elevate HOB to 30 to 45° with minimized activity if increased ICP suspected.

2. Institute all safety measures by elevating side rails, and padding side rails if client restless or disoriented.

3. Apply ice bag to back of neck or forehead during headache episodes, and to side of neck with vomiting episodes.

4. Apply O_2 at 2 L/min by nasal cannula if respirations become shallow or labored.

5. Orient to time, place, and reason for hospitalization with each client contact when changes in LOC occur.

6. Place call light and personal articles within easy reach and instruct client in their location.

7. Use a slow, deliberate, and low pitched voice when communicating with client.

8. Passive ROME to all major joints 3 times a day q 8 hr if tolerated.

9. Mouth care using soft toothbrush and oral antiseptic q 8 hr and after all vomiting episodes. Once a day, clean teeth with a mixture of H_2O_2 and baking soda.

10. Offer bedpan or urinal q 4 hr and record time and amount of all incontinences.

11. Assist client to perform all ADLs and maintain judicious independence over self and environment with physical limitations.

12. Back care and massage to all bony prominences using lotion q 4 hr while on bedrest.

13. Instruct client and family on
Ways to eliminate Valsalva maneuver: no straining, coughing, holding breath, or sneezing
Purpose of ICP monitoring using terms appropriate to client's learning level
Reason for elevated side rails
Reason for fluid restriction if appropriate

Change–Interdependent

1. Notify physician if:
Changes in LOC or behavior occurs
Headache or seizures occur
Pupil size becomes unequal or fixed
Systolic BP elevates with widening pulse pressure
Bradycardia occurs
Respiratory pattern changes
Changes in vision, gait, and speech occur in addition to other indications of increased ICP

2. Medicate appropriately for headache, vomiting, seizures, and assess effect in 10 to 20 min.

3. Cleanse ICP monitoring insertion site with betadine solution and cover with a dry sterile dressing qd.

4. Anticipate physician to prescribe:
ICP monitoring to determine increases in pressure

Lasix: 60 to 80 mg IV push
Decadron: up to 100 mg/24 hr
Mannitol: 20% 2 g/kg body weight IV push
Glycerol: 1 g/kg body weight by NG tube
Fluid restriction to 1500 ml/24 hr with onset of cerebral edema
Whole brain radiation with multiple metastasis—2000 rads per week to
    4000 rads in 3 weeks
Ventriculostomy to relieve pressure if other measures fail

BIBLIOGRAPHY

Breunig, K.A. After the blowup...How to care for the patient with a ruptured cerebral aneurysm. *Nursing 76*, 1976, 37–45.
Conway-Rutkowksi, B.L. *Carini and Owen's neurological and neurosurgical nursing* (8th ed.). St. Louis: C.V. Mosby, 1982.
Corbett, J.V. *Laboratory tests in nursing practice.* Norwalk, Connecticut: Appleton-Century-Crofts, 1982.
Gordon, M. *Manual of nursing diagnosis.* New York: McGraw-Hill, 1982.
Ryan, L.S. Nursing assessment of the ambulatory patient with brain metastases. *Cancer Nursing*, 4(4), 1981, 281–291.
Shapiro, W.R. Life-threatening neurological complications of cancer. *Current Problems in Cancer* (Vol. 4, No. 3.). Chicago: Year Book Medical, 1979, pp. 83–85.
Wilson, C.B. Fulton, D.S., and Seager, M.L. Supportive management of the patient with malignant brain tumor. *Journal of the American Medical Association*, 244(11), 1980, 1249–1251.

30. Spinal Cord Compression

DEFINITION AND CAUSATIVE FACTORS

Spinal cord compression in the client with cancer results from malignancies that originate from spinal column structures or from metastasis to the vertebrae. Spinal lesions are classified according to location as intradural, extradural, and extravertebral. Extravertebral tumors extend through the vertebral foramen and partially involve the spinal cord. Extradural tumors do not involve the cord, but develop in areas between the periosteum and the dura causing destruction to the vertebral bodies, laminae, pedicles, and epidural tissues. Metastatic spinal involvement is usually extradural. Intradural extramedullary tumors occur within the dura, meninges, ligaments, or nerve roots. Intradural intramedullary tumors originate within the spinal cord itself and constitute only 5% of all spinal cord tumors.

Fifteen percent of spinal cord compressions are located in the cervical spine, 68% are thoracic, and 16% are lumbosacral. Malignant spinal cord involvement develops through the venous pathway of the paravertebral and extradural venous plexus by direct invasion of lymph into the epidural space and by bony erosion from direct extension of the malignancy. Pain is the most common symptom; other manifestations include motor and sensory deficits which vary according to location and structural involvement of the tumor. Laminectomy with spinal fusion and/or radiation are the recommended therapies.

Corresponding metastic cancers (extradural) are in order of incidence:

- Cervical spine—lung, breast, melanoma, lymphoma, kidney, and myeloma
- Thoracic spine—lung, breast, kidney, prostate, lymphoma, myeloma, melanoma, and GI
- Lumbosacral spine—GI, melanoma, lymphoma, myeloma, kidney, prostate, breast, and lung
- Corresponding intradural and extravertebral cancers are:
  Intradural intramedullary—ependymous, astrocytoma, and gliomas
  Intradural extramedullary—neurilemmona, meningioma
  Extravertebral—lymphoma, seminoma, neuroblastoma

ASSESSMENT DATA

- Pain—local (neck, back, lumbar)
  Gradual at first
  Worse with Valsalva maneuver and motion
  Aggravated with supine position, relieved with sitting position
  Intense vertebral collapse
- Pain—radicular (root)
  Related to distribution of segmental dermatome
  Aggravated by movement
  Often misinterpreted as other conditions (e.g., T-7 root as ulcers, T-8 as gallbladder)
- Pain—medullary
  Diffuse or referred pain (not radicular)
  Usually bilateral
  Shooting or burning in peripheral areas
  Not aggravated by Valsalva maneuver
- Motor deficits
  Weakness
  Ataxia
  Extremities feel tired or heavy
  Damage to corticospinal tract—spasticity, spastic paralysis, hyperreflexia, positive Babinski
  Damage to lower motor neurons—hypotonicity, flaccid paralysis, hyporeflexia, atrophy
- Sensory deficits
  Damage to spinothalamic tracts—loss of pain and temperature sensation
  Damage to dorsal columns—paresthesia
  Central cord syndrome—motor loss greater in arms than legs with varying sensory loss caused by edema, tumor, or hemorrhage interrupting the blood supply to the spinal cord
  Anterior cord syndrome—motor loss (paralysis) with intact sensory function
  Brown–Sequard syndrome—caused by a lesion on lateral portion of spinal cord involving one-half of the cord resulting in weakness in the side of the lesion, and diminished pain and temperature on the opposite side
  Spinal shock—usually follows a complete spinal cord transection but may also occur with an incomplete spinal cord lesion—loss of motor, sensory, autonomic and reflex function below the level of the lesion
  Paraplegia—if it occurs before surgery, it is usually irreversible
  Respiratory arrest can occur if C 1-3 are severely involved
  Autonomic dysfunction of bowel and bladder—retention or incontinence

Spinal x-rays—erosion or calcification of spine

Lumbar puncture—Quekenstadt sign, partial or complete block when jugular veins manually compressed. CSF may be yellow with spontaneous coagulation and increased protein.

Myelogram—outlines location of tumor and degree of block

Electromyography—demonstrates fasciculations and denervation from motor nerve root compression

NURSING DIAGNOSES

RATIONALE

Alteration in comfort level, acute pain, related to destruction of the spinal column and damage to the cord and spinal nerve roots, resulting from spinal cord compression.

Direct neural pressure or interference with circulation.

Associated Nursing Diagnoses

1. Impaired physical mobility, related to upper or lower motor neuron damage, resulting in muscle weakness, reflex alterations, or paralysis.

Lack of continuous tonic discharges from higher centers to the cord neurons.

2. Sensory deficit, uncompensated, related to damage to the spinothalamic tracts, resulting in loss of pain and temperature.

Pain signals cross at the anterior commissure in the spine and pass up toward the brain via the anterolateral spinothalamic pathway. Temperature is regulated by nervous feedback mechanisms associated with the spinal cord.

3. Alteration in bowel and urinary elimination (increased or decreased), related to a disruption of innervation to the sigmoid colon, bladder, and sphincters, resulting in loss of control of elimination.

The bladder is innervated at the external sphincter, bladder neck, trigone, and detrusor muscle. The defecation reflex is enhanced by innervation of the internal and external sphincters, rectum, sigmoid, and descending colon.

4. Impaired skin integrity, related to surgical intervention to decompress the spinal cord.

Laminectomy requires a midline incision in the back over the spinous processes of the vertebrae.

NURSING INTERVENTIONS

Monitoring–Independent

1. Assess client for pain with each contact and record:
   Location
   Intensity—at rest, with movement, or Valsalva
   Radiation—unilateral or bilateral
   Duration—constant or intermittent
   Character—shooting, burning, dull, or sharp
   Aggravating and alleviating factors
2. Inspect muscles of arms and legs q 8 hr and record presence or onset of:
   Atrophy
   Fasciculations
   Involuntary movements
   Lack of voluntary movement
   Abnormal positions
3. Test client's muscle strength in arms by hand grip and in legs by pushing feet against resistance q 8 hr and record by grade 0 to 5 (5 = normal).
4. Test client's coordination by touching each finger with thumb and by tapping nurse's hand with ball of each foot q 8 hr.
5. Test client for sensory function q 8 hr and record abnormal responses for:
   Pain—sharp or dull sensations with safety pin
   Temperature—cold, warm sensations using hot or cold water filled test tubes
   Light touch—using cotton
   Vibration—using tuning fork over joints
   Position—ask client to describe position of a limb in space
6. Test appropriate or selected reflexes q 8 hr and record grade 0 to +4 (+2 = normal).
   Biceps: C-5, C-6
   Triceps: C-7, C-8
   Upper abdominal: T-8, T-9, T-10 (stroking causes muscle contraction)
   Lower abdominal: T-10, T-11, T-12
   Knee: L-2, L-3, L-4
   Ankle: S-1, S-2
   Plantar (Babinski): L-4, L-5, S-1, S-2
7. BP, heart rate, and respirations q 15 to 30 min if client in spinal shock, or postoperatively until stable, q 2 to 4 hr otherwise.
8. Assess LOC q 1 hr with spinal shock or postoperatively, q 4 to 8 hr otherwise.
9. Assess skin color, temperature, and moisture q 2 to 4 hr.

10. Auscultate breath sounds in all lung fields q 1 hr during critical phase, q 4 to 8 hr thereafter.
11. Assess symmetry of chest expansion, depth of respirations, and use of accessory muscles q 1 hr or q 4 to 8 hr.
12. Assess pupils for size and bilateral reaction to light q 2 to 4 hr.
13. Auscultate bowel sounds in 4 quadrants q 4 to 8 hr and record onset and location of changes in pitch and frequency.
14. Temperature q 4 hr.
15. Palpate peripheral pulses for bilateral quality q 8 hr.
16. Inspect dependent areas for edema q 8 hr.
17. Auscultate heart sounds in 4 valvular sites q 8 hr and record changes in rate and rhythm.
18. Palpate bladder distention q 2 hr. Calculate fullness from last voiding by 30 to 60 ml × number of hours = expected volume. (30 to 60 ml represents the minimum amount of urine produced by the kidneys in 1 hr.)
19. Accurate I and O, calculate I/O ratio for fluid balance q 8 and 24 hr.
20. Inspect surgical dressing postoperatively q 4 hr and record amount and color of drainage.

Monitoring–Interdependent

1. Assess entry sites of cervical skeletal traction (if applicable) q 8 hr for redness, pain, swelling, or exudate formation.
2. Assess traction for rope integrity alignment, and correct poundage of weights q 8 hr.
3. Assess results of laboratory data when available and compare to previous or normal values:
   Routine preoperative
   CBC   Hemoglobin: 13.0 to 18.0 g/dl males
                     12.0 to 16.0 g/dl females
         Hematocrit: 45 to 52% males
                     37 to 48% females
        RBC: 4.6 to 6.2 × 10^6/mm^3 males
            4.2 to 5.4 × 10^6/mm^3 females
       WBC: 4,500 to 11,500/mm^3
       Platelets: 130,000 to 370,000 mm^3
   Urinalysis: Negative for RBC, WBC, protein, sugar, and acetone
   Serum Sodium: 135 to 145 mEq/L
   Serum Potassium: 3.5 to 5.0 mEq/L
   Serum Chloride: 100 to 106 mEq/L
   Serum Calcium: 8.5 to 10.5 mg/dl
   Blood Sugar: 70 to 100 mg/dl

Change–Independent

1. Maintain bedrest with onset of back pain and/or motor or sensory deficits.
2. Position client with maximum comfort and maintain body alignment using sandbags and pillows.
3. Apply O_2 at 2 L/min by nasal cannula with onset of respiratory distress.
4. Offer bedpan or urinal every 2 hr.
5. Offer 120 ml of po fluids (if applicable) alternating with fat free milk and juice of choice q 2 hr while awake.
6. Cough and deep breathe q 4 hr.
7. Back care and deep massage with lotion to all bony prominences q 4 hr.
8. Passive ROME to all extremities while maintaining strict body alignment q 4 hr.
9. Turn from side, to back, to side using log rolling technique q 4 hr.
10. Mouth care q 4 hr with oral antiseptic of choice. Once a day, clean teeth with a mixture of H_2O_2 and baking soda to neutralize oral acid and remove plaque.
11. Assist client to perform ADLs and maintain judicious independence and control over self and environment within physical limitations.
12. Institute all safety measures by elevating side rails and arranging call light and personal articles within reach.
13. Explain condition and progress to client and family with each contact. Assist them to ask questions and express concerns of the present and the future.
14. Include family members in plan of care and allow them to participate, if mutually therapeutic.

Change–Interdependent

1. Medicate for pain as prescribed and assess effect in 5 to 20 min.
2. Notify physician if:
    Onset or increase in severity of local or radicular pain occurs
    Onset of paralysis or other motor and sensory deficits occur
    Systolic blood pressure less than 90 torr
    Heart rate less than 50 beats per min
    Respiratory distress develops
    Temperature elevation greater than 101.0° F occurs (especially just before or after surgery)
    Bowel or bladder retention occurs. Be alert for signs of autonomic dysreflexia.

3. Anticipate physician to prescribe:
Laminectomy and/or radiation (3000 to 4000 rads over 2 to 8 wk) to decompress the spinal cord
Dexamethasone (Decadron): 100 mg for 3 days to control edema prior to surgery
Spinal cord cooling (local hypothermia) to reduce cord injury from edema. Under anesthesia, iced saline is pumped into the spinal canal by a perfusion circuit for 3 hr
Systemic chemotherapy
Microsurgical removal of intradural intramedullary tumors
Cervical fractures—skeletal traction (Crutchfield, Barton, Garder-Wells, or Vinke tongs) with Stryker frame, Foster frame or CircOlectric bed

BIBLIOGRAPHY

Arsenault, L. Primary spinal cord tumors: A review and case presentation of a patient with an intramedullary spinal cord neoplasm. *Journal of Neurosurgical Nursing*, 13(2), 1981, 53–58.
Bates, B. *A guide to physical examination* (3rd ed.). Philadelphia: J. B. Lippincott, 1983.
Cairncross, J.G., and Posner, J.B. Neurological complications of systemic cancer—Spinal cord compression. In J. Yarbro and R. Bornstein (Eds.), *Oncologic emergencies*. New York: Grune and Stratton, 1981, pp. 82–87.
Carabell, S.C., and Goodman, R.L. Spinal cord compression. In V.T. DeVita, S. Hellman, and S.A. Rosenberg (Eds.), *Cancer, principles and practice of oncology*. Philadelphia: J.B. Lippincott, 1982, pp. 1589–1593.
Corbett, J.V. *Laboratory tests in nursing practice*. Norwalk, Connecticut: Appleton-Century-Crofts, 1982.
Davis, J.E., and Mason, C.B. *Neurological critical care*. New York: Van Nostrand Reinhold, 1979.
Donoghue, M. Spinal cord compression. In J.M. Yasko (Ed.), *Guidelines for cancer care—Symptom management*. Reston, Virginia: Reston, 1983, pp. 353–357.
Gordon, M. *Manual of nursing diagnosis*. New York: McGraw-Hill, 1982.
Luckman, J., and Sorensen, K.C. *Medical-surgical nursing—A psychophysiologic approach* (2nd ed.). Philadelphia: W.B. Saunders, 1980.
McOuat, F. The insidious spinal cord tumor. *Journal of Neurosurgical Nursing*, 13(1), 1981, 18–22.
Swift-Bandini, N. *Manual of neurological nursing* (2nd ed.). Boston: Little, Brown, 1982.

31. Meningeal Carcinomatosis

DEFINITION AND CAUSATIVE FACTORS

Meningeal carcinomatosis occurs when tumor cells infiltrate the arachnoid and pia mater (leptomeninges) of the cerebrum, cerebellum, and spinal cord causing diffuse or multifocal involvement on the surfaces of these structures. Direct invasion of the parenchyma may or may not develop, and it can occur months or years after successful cancer treatment. The dissemination of the cancer cells to the leptomeninges is thought to be blood borne, along nerve roots, tumors of the parenchyma, or by way of the choroid plexus. The incidence of meningeal carcinomatosis is increasing most probably as a result of greater awareness and increased survival rates. The symptoms vary depending on the site of infiltration—cerebral, cranial, or spinal—but the most serious complication involves the blockade of CSF in the subarachnoid space causing increased intracranial pressure with hydrocephalus, uncal herniation, and death. Systemic chemotherapy is unsuccessful in the treatment of meningeal carcinomatosis because most of these drugs do not cross the blood–brain barrier. Direct ventricular infusion of Methotrexate using an Ommaya reservoir and craniospinal radiation is the preferred therapy. Diagnosis is made by CSF analysis, myelogram, and CT scan.

CSF pressure is increased in 64% of clients, protein is increased in 85%, and glucose is decreased in 65%. Both CSF protein and glucose are normal in 10% of clients.

Corresponding cancers include non-Hodgkin lymphoma (histiocytic), acute leukemias, breast, lung, bronchogenic tumors, gastric, prostate, pancreas, Hodgkin, and melanoma.

ASSESSMENT DATA

- Cerebral
  Headache and stiff neck without temperature elevation
  Change in LOC
  Lethargy
  Memory loss

- Cranial
    Diplopia, blurred vision
    Dysarthria
    Hearing deficit
- Spinal
    Muscle weakness
    Back pain
    Bowel and bladder incontinence
    Paresthesia
    Ataxia
- Increased intracranial pressure (ICP)
    Restlessness
    Decreased LOC
    Widening pulse pressure with increasing systolic BP
    Bradycardia
    Change in respirations
    Nausea and vomiting
    Dilated pupils (first unilateral, then bilateral)
    CSF pressure—increased
    CSF analysis (multiple taps required)
        Increased protein content
        Increased WBC
        Decreased glucose
    CT scan—blurred cranial borders with hydrocephalus
    Myelogram—irregular nerve roots and defective filling of subarach-
        noid space

NURSING DIAGNOSES

*Alteration in tissue perfusion re-
lated to a blockade of CSF causing
hydrocephalus, uncal herniation,
and death.*

RATIONALE

*The brain, CSF, and blood volume
are confined to a nonexpandable
space (skull). Any increase in these
structures causes increased ICP
and neurological deficits.*

Associated Nursing Diagnoses

1. Alteration in comfort level,
   acute, pain, related to headache
   and back pain, resulting from
   increased intracranial pressure
   or spinal meningeal metastasis.

Obstruction of CSF by tumor raises
intracranial pressure. Compression of spinal nerves by tumor
load results in back pain.

2. Sensory deficit, uncompensated, related to visual, tactile,
   and hearing disturbances, resulting from a neurologic
   impairment.

Sensory information from body re-
   ceptors is altered due to various
   synaptic functions of neurons.

3. Alteration in bowel and urinary
   elimination, related to spinal
   metastasis interrupting the
   sensory and motor pathways involving control of elimination.

Uninhibited neurogenic bladder
   due to a defect in the corticoreg-
   ulatory tracts with symptoms of
   increased frequency, urgency,
   and incontinence. Autonomous
   neurogenic bladder seen in neoplasms involving the conus
   medullaris, cauda equina, or
   pelvic nerves.

Bowel complications result from
   impaired level of consciousness
   or intestinal tumor obstruction.

4. Potential for infection related to
   the Ommaya reservoir which
   introduces a potential pathway
   for bacterial contamination of
   the ventricle

Intraventricular cannula creates access port for infection.

NURSING INTERVENTIONS

Monitoring–Independent

1. Assess LOC with each client contact and record onset of changes in
   awareness, orientation, and behavior.
2. Assess client for headache (throbbing, pulsating, aggravated by a change
   to an upright position or due to sneezing or coughing), stiff neck, and
   back pain with each contact.
3. Inspect bilateral pupil responses q 2 hr for:
   Direct light reflex
   Consensual light reflex
   Sluggish or brisk reaction
   Accommodation—convergence and constriction
   Size and quality of pupil size
4. Assess visual acuity by asking client to read aloud a short printed passage
   q 6 hr and record subjective complaints of blurred vision.
5. Assess hearing acuity by asking client to perform simple commands in
   varying voice volumes q 6 hr and record changes.

6. BP, heart rate, respirations q 1 hr with indications of increased ICP and record pulse pressure and onset of changes in respiratory and heart rate.

7. Assess client for nausea with each contact and record number of emesis episodes.

8. Accurate I and O and calculate I/O ratio for fluid balance q 8 and 24 hr.

9. Test client's ability to move extremities on command and respond appropriately to deep and light touch stimuli q 8 hr.

10. Test muscle strength in extremities by firmness of hand grip and ability to push hand away with foot using counterforce q 8 hr.

11. Assess client for activity tolerance and steady gait with each contact and record subjective indications of weakness or fatigue.

12. Assess client for bowel and bladder dysfunction with each contact.

13. Record onset of difficult or absent speech.

14. Assess client for seizure activity with each contact.

15. Temperature q 4 hr.

16. Inspect oral cavity for stomatitis q 8 hr with MTX chemotherapy.

Monitoring–Interdependent

1. Assess results of laboratory data when available and compare to previous and normal values.

    CSF   Pressure: 100 to 200 torr
            Protein: 20 to 45 mg %
            Glucose: 50 to 100 mg %
    CT Scan indicating meningeal carcinomatosis
    Myelogram indicating meningeal carcinomatosis

2. Assess insertion site of Ommaya reservoir for pain, redness, leakage, or swelling 8 q hr.

Change–Independent

1. Maintain bedrest and elevate HOB to 30 to 45° with minimized activity if increased ICP suspected.

2. Institute all safety measures by elevating side rails, and padding side rails if client restless or disoriented.

3. Apply ice bag to back of neck or forehead during headache episodes, and to side of neck with vomiting episodes.

4. Apply O_2 at 2 L/min by nasal cannula if respirations become shallow or labored.

5. Orient to time, place, and reason for hospitalization with each client contact when changes in LOC occur.

6. Place call light and personal articles within easy reach and instruct client in their location.
7. Use a slow, deliberate, low pitched voice when communicating with client.
8. Passive ROME to all major joints 3 times a day if tolerated.
9. Offer bedpan or urinal q 4 hr and record time and amount of all incontinences.
10. Assist client to perform all ADLs and maintain judicious independence over self and environment within physical limitations.
11. Instruct client and family:
     To notify nurse for assistance with all ambulating needs.
     Ways to eliminate Valsalva maneuver: no straining, holding breath, or coughing, sneezing
     Purpose of the Ommaya reservoir, signs of infection, and avoidance of head trauma using terms appropriate to client's learning level
     Reason for elevated side rails
     Reason for restricted po fluids, if applicable
     Transfer techniques if appropriate
12. Mouth care after meals and at hour of sleep using soft toothbrush and $\frac{1}{2}$ strength H_2O_2. Once a day, clean teeth with a mixture of H_2O_2 and baking soda to neutralize oral acid and remove plaque.
13. Passive ROME q 4 hr to all extremities while on bedrest.
14. Reposition and deep breathe q 2 hr.
15. Back care q 4 hr and massage all bony prominences with lotion.
16. Institute seizure precautions—oral airway and padded tongue blade at bedside; if seizure occurs, remove all environmental hazards, loosen constrictive clothing around neck, support head and turn to one side to allow tongue to fall forward, and do NOT restrain.

Change–Interdependent

1. Notify physician if:
     Headache and stiff neck occur
     Pupil size becomes unequal or fixed
     Changes in vision, hearing, gait, and activity tolerance occur in addition to other indications of increased ICP
     Temperature elevation greater than 101.0° F
     Change in LOC occurs
     Systolic BP elevated with widening pulse pressure
     Respiratory pattern changes
     Bradycardia occurs
     Seizure activity occurs
     Methotrexate side effects occur—headache, fever, encephalopathy

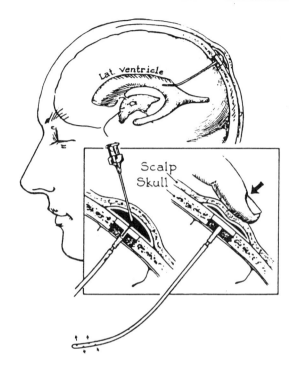

Figure 31-1. The Ommaya reservoir. Source: Ommaya, A., and Ratcheson, R., Experience with the subcutaneous CSF reservoir. New England Journal of Medicine, **279**,(19), 1968, 1026, with permission.

2. Medicate appropriately for headache, seizure activity, temperature elevation, and nausea, and assess effect in 10 to 20 min.

3. Cleanse Ommaya reservoir insertion site with betadine solution and cover with dry sterile dressing qd.

4. Anticipate physician to prescribe:

Intrathecal or intraventricular chemotherapy

Ommaya reservoir insertion (Fig. 31-1)*

Methotrexate: 6.25 to 10.0 mg/m^2 body surface, twice a week until spinal fluid clear. Use of leucovorin rescue must be delayed 12 to 24 hr following intrathecal or intraventricular MTX as leucovorin rapidly enters the CSF.

Cytosine arabinoside chemotherapy may also be used.

Radiation—whole brain for cerebral and cranial involvement with 3,000 to 4,000 rads, 1200 to 2000 rads for spinal involvement

Mannitol 20% 500 ml or by bolus 50 to 100 g *and*

Dexamethasone (Decadron) 6 to 10 mg q 6 hr *and*

---

*A silastic dome inserted in scalp with a catheter extending into lateral ventricle which can also be used for ventricular drainage, instillation of antibiotics and chemotherapy, and CSF analysis. Complications include infection and seizures.

Furosemide (Lasix) 60 to 80 mg *and*
Fluid restriction to 1500 ml/24 hr for increased ICP from edema
Antiemetic, anticonvulsant, and analgesic medications
Foley indwelling catheter
Stool softeners

BIBLIOGRAPHY

Bates, B. *A guide to physical examination* (3rd ed.). Philadelphia: J.B. Lippincott, 1983.
Corbett, J.V. *Laboratory tests in nursing practice.* Norwalk, Connecticut: Appleton-Century-Crofts, 1982.
Fulton, D.S., et al. Intrathecal cytosine arabinoside for the treatment of meningeal metastases from malignant brain tumors and systemic tumors. *Cancer Chemotherapy and Pharmacology,* **8**, 1982, 285–291.
Gargen, R. Nursing management of the patient with meningeal carcinomatosis. *Journal of Neurosurgical Nursing,* **12**(4), 1980, 184–186.
Gordon, M. *Manual of nursing diagnosis.* New York: McGraw-Hill, 1982.
Horton, J., and Hill, G.J. *Clinical oncology.* Philadelphia: W.B. Saunders, 1977.
Luckman, J., and Sorensen, K.C. *Medical–surgical nursing—A psychophysiologic approach* (2nd ed.). Philadelphia: W.B. Saunders, 1980.
Mehta, B.M., Glass, J.P., and Shapiro, W.R. Serum and cerebrospinal fluid distribution of 5-methyltetrahydrofolate after intravenous calcium leucovorin and intra-Ommaya methotrexate administration in patients with meningeal carcinomatosis. *Cancer Research,* **43**, 1983, 435–438.
Portlock, C.S., and Goffinet, D.R. *Manual of clinical problems in oncology.* Boston: Little, Brown, 1980.
Shapiro, W.R. Life-threatening neurological complications of cancer. *Current Problems in Cancer* (Vol. 4, No. 3.). Chicago: Year Book Medical, 1979, pp. 77–80.
Swift-Bandini, N. *Manual of neurological nursing* (2nd ed.). Boston: Little, Brown, 1982.
Wujcik, D. Meningeal carcinomatosis: Diagnosis, treatment, and nursing care. *Oncology Nursing Forum,* **10**(2), 1983, 35–40.

PART VII
INTEGUMENT

32. Chemotherapy Related Extravasation

DEFINITION AND CAUSATIVE FACTORS

Extravasation is the escape of a vesicant (blistering) or sclerosing (scarring) chemotherapeutic agent from the venipuncture site into the surrounding tissues causing inflammation, ulceration, and/or necrosis. This damage can involve not only the subcutaneous tissues but muscles, nerves, tendons, and blood vessels located in the area. When ulceration occurs, skin grafting may be necessary. The amount of infiltration, area involved, and length of exposure to the agent will determine the extent of cellular damage. Central venous catheters, single (Fig. 32-1) or double lumen (Fig. 32-2), can reduce the incidence of extravasation. Table 32-1 lists some of the chemotherapeutic drugs and tissue reactions to extravasation, and Table 32-2 provides antidotes proven effective in minimizing or preventing tissue damage.

Corresponding cancers associated with chemotherapy related extravasation include all those treated with vesicant or sclerosing chemotherapeutic drugs (Table 32-3).

Previously used IV sites, inflammation, large bore IV needles, tissue trauma in area of IV site, inadequate dilution of drug, prior radiation of site, sclerotic vascular disease, and venous obstruction due to lymphedema or lymph node dissection are additional causes.

ASSESSMENT DATA

- No blood return from IV
- Redness and inflammation at site
- Burning at site
- Warmth at site
- Edema at site or proximal to insertion site
- Phlebitis
- Pain at site

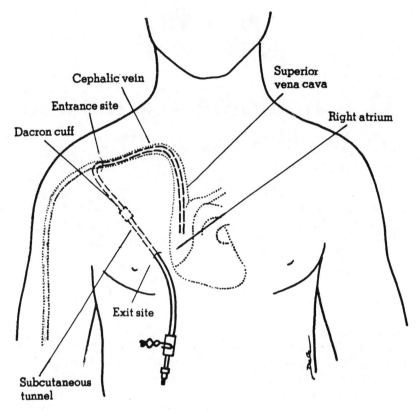

Figure 32-1. Placement of the single lumen Hickman catheter. A 2-inch incision is made in the deltopectoral groove below the acromion of the right clavicle, and the cephalic vein is isolated. Then, a subcutaneous tunnel is formed using long forceps, exiting at an area between the sternum and the nipple. The catheter is pulled through the tunnel, inserted in the cephalic vein, and positioned in the lower superior vena cava at the entrance to the right atrium. The Dacron cuff is positioned in the subcutaneous tunnel. The tunnel and the cuff serve as barriers to infection. Source: Bjeletich, J., and Hickman, R.O., 1980, with permission.

NURSING DIAGNOSES

Potential impairment of skin integrity, related to IV administration of vesicant or sclerosing chemotherapy and the hazard of infiltration, resulting in extravasation.

RATIONALE

Chemotherapeutic agents with an acidic pH may cause cellular tissue damage.

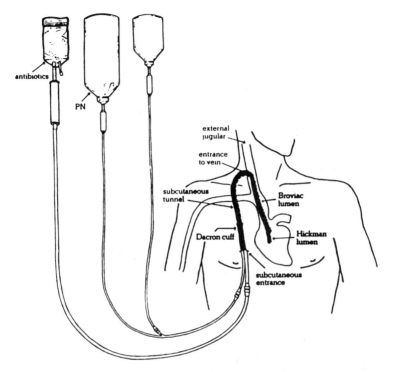

Figure 32-2. Placement of the double lumen Hickman catheter. Source: Anderson, M.A., Aker, S.N., and Hickman, R.O., 1982, with permission.

Associated Nursing Diagnoses

1. Alteration of comfort level, related to the acute pain associated with infiltration of chemotherapeutic agents, resulting in extravasation.

   Cellular tissue breakdown increases nerve stimulation by direct access or indirect access, such as compression due to inflammation and edema.

2. Potential for physical injury to muscle, nerve, tendon, and blood vessel tissue, related to inflammation, necrosis, and ulceration from vesicant or sclerosing agents, resulting in extravasation.

   Degree of physical injury is directly proportional to the amount of the acidic drug absorbed, the length of exposure and the area involved.

TABLE 32-1. VESICANT ANTICANCER DRUGS AND THEIR CLINICAL MANIFESTATIONS

Drug	Type of Reaction	Onset of Inflammation	Symptoms	Duration of Reaction	Mechanism
Carmustine	Vein phlebitis	10–14 days	Pain	7 days	Endothelial alkylation
Dactinomycin	Vesicant, recall	1–2 weeks	Pain	Several weeks	Inhibition of DNA-directed RNA synthesis
Daunorubicin	Vesicant	1–2 weeks	Pain	Several weeks	Tissue DNA intercalation superoxide formation
Doxorubicin	Vesicant, recall	1–2 weeks	Pain	Several weeks	Tissue DNA intercalation superoxide formation
Fluorouracil	Discoloration	1 week	No pain	1 week	Unknown
Mechlorethamine	Vesicant	12–24 hours	Pain	4–6 weeks	Tissue alkylation
	Vein discoloration	2 weeks	No pain	3–4 weeks	Endothelial alkylation
Mithramycin	Vesicant	1 week	Pain	Several weeks	Tissue alkylation
Mitomycin C	Vesicant	1 week	Pain	Several weeks	Tissue alkylation superoxide formation
Vinblastine	Vesicant	12–24 hours	Pain	Several weeks	Mitotic inhibition
Vincristine	Vesicant	12–24 hours	Pain	Several weeks	Mitotic inhibition

(Source: See-Lasley, K., Ignoffo, R. J., 1981, with permission.)

TABLE 32-2. ANTIDOTES FOR VESICANT CANCER DRUGS

Drug	Antidote	Dose
	Manufacturer recommended	
Mechlorethamine	Sodium thiosulfate 10%	4 ml
Vincristine	Heat + hyaluronidase (150 μ/ml)	150 units
	Theoretical	
Actinomycin C	Sodium thiosulfate 10%	4 ml
	or	
	Ascorbic acid injection (50 mg/ml)	1 ml
Carmustine	Sodium bicarbonate 8.4%	5 ml
Daunorubicin	Sodium bicarbonate 8.4% plus	5 ml
	dexamethasone 4 mg/ml	1 ml
Doxorubicin	Sodium bicarbonate 8.4% plus	5 ml
	dexamethasone 4 mg/ml	1 ml
Mithramycin	EDTA 150 mg/ml	1 ml
Mitomycin C	Sodium thiosulfate 10%	4 ml
	or	
	Ascorbic acid 50 mg/ml	1 ml
	or	
	Pyridoxine HCl 50 mg/ml	1 ml
Vinblastine	Sodium bicarbonate 8.4%	5 ml
	or	
	Heat + hyaluronidase (150 μ/ml)	150 units

(Source: from See-Lasley, K., and Ignoffo, R. J., 1981, with permission.)

NURSING INTERVENTIONS

Monitoring–Interdependent

1. Assess type of chemotherapeutic agent(s) (vesicant, sclerosing [Table 32-1], recommended dilution, infusion rate, and infusion method prior to administration).
2. Assess IV arm for swelling, inflammation, previously used IV sites, including veins utilized for recent laboratory work, and other tissue trauma proximal to IV insertion site prior to peripheral chemotherapy administration.
3. Assess patency of IV by injecting 10 ml saline and observe for infiltration at insertion site and along vein tract proximal to insertion site prior to and following each peripheral chemotherapy administration.
4. Aspirate for blood return prior to peripheral chemotherapy administration and after every 3 ml of chemotherapy if IV pushed.
5. Assess insertion site of central venous catheter for drainage, redness, and swelling prior to central chemotherapy administration.
6. Aspirate for blood return from central venous catheter.

TABLE 32-3. CHEMOTHERAPEUTIC AGENTS RELATED TO EXTRAVASATION

Dactinomycin (Actinomycin-D), (Cosmegen)	Mechlorethamine hydrochloride (Nitrogen Mustard), (Mustargen)
Doxorubicin hydrochloride (Adriamycin)	Platinum (Cis-Platinum)
Vindesine (DAVA)	Streptozocin (Streptozotocin)
Daunorubicin hydrochloride (Daunomycin)	Vinblastine sulfate (Velban)
6-Mercaptopurine (6-MP) (Purinethol)	Vincristine sulfate (Oncovin)
Mithramycin (Mithracin)	Carmustine (BCNU)
Mitomycin C (Mutamycin)	Dacarbazine (DTIC)

7. Assess area of insertion site and area surrounding peripheral vein tract for swelling and inflammation q 5 to 10 min ✕4 and q 30 min thereafter with slow infusions; immediately with IV push administration and q 3 min ✕5.
8. Assess client for generalized adverse reactions—temperature elevation, skin rash or urticaria, SOB or dyspnea, tachycardia, and edema, during and for 1 hr after chemotherapy administration (See Chapter 25).
9. Assess all areas of previous extravasation for inflammation, ulceration, and necrosis qd.

Change–Independent

1. Teach client (if appropriate):
   Name and action of chemotherapeutic agent(s)
   Potential side effects
   To report burning or swelling at insertion site during chemotherapy administration
   To report nausea, vomiting, feeling hot, itching, and trouble breathing during chemotherapy administration, and up to 3 hours post-administration
2. Assess IV for secure placement q 8 hr if client is ambulatory or active.
3. Provide diversional activities depending on client's interest during chemotherapy administration.

Change–Interdependent

1. Use recommended dilution of chemotherapeutic agent according to manufacturer or agency protocol.
2. Use 20 or 21 gauge IV needle. Avoid IV administration of vesicant drugs in hand, wrist, or over joints.
3. Remove all constricting tape proximal to IV insertion site.

4. Change IV site if:

   Area proximal to IV insertion site has any evidence of swelling, inflammation, or trauma

   Old venipuncture sites are located proximal to present IV site

   Saline injection demonstrates infiltration into tissues or leakage around entry

   Blood return absent or present but difficult to withdraw, contains bubbles, or dilute

   Client complains of burning along IV tract

5. If extravasation should occur (or according to protocol):

   Stop infusion

   Aspirate up to 5 ml of blood

   Using a 25 or 27 gauge IV needle, aspirate infiltration area to remove as much extravasated solution as possible

   Inject 25 mg hydrocortisone into infiltrated tissue subcutaneously or directly through the IV or antidote according to Table 32-2

   Remove needle and cover site with dry sterile dressing

   Apply ice to area if Adriamycin (Doxorubicin) infiltrates

   Apply ice for 1 hr, then heat for 1 hr, cold for 1 hr, and heat for 6 hr for all other agents

6. Change dressing on central venous catheter insertion site qd. Cleanse the site using half strength H_2O_2 followed by betadine, and betadine ointment and cover with clear plastic, sterile adhesive (Op-Site) or according to agency protocol.

7. Anticipate physician to surgically excise areas of ulceration and necrosis.

8. Notify physician if:

   Extravasation should occur

   Ulceration develops

   Systemic indications of anaphylaxis occur

   Infection occurs as evidenced by temperature elevation greater than 101° F and WBC greater than 12,000/mm^3

BIBLIOGRAPHY

Anderson, M.A., Aker, S.N., and Hickman, R.O. The double lumen Hickman catheter. *American Journal of Nursing*, 82(2), 1982, 272–273.

Barlock, A.L., Howser, D.M., and Hubbard, S.M. Nursing management of adriamycin extravasation. *American Journal of Nursing*, 79(1), 1979, 94–96.

Bjeletich, J., and Hickman, R.O. The Hickman indwelling catheter. *American Journal of Nursing*, 80(1), 1980, 62–65.

Gordon, M. *Manual of nursing diagnosis*. New York: McGraw-Hill, 1982.

Lauffer, B. Extravasation. In J.M. Yasko (Ed.), *Guidelines for cancer care—Symptom management*. Virginia: Reston, 1983, pp. 330–335.

See-Lasley, K., and Ignoffo, R.J. *Manual of oncology therapeutics*. St. Louis: C. V. Mosby, 1981, pp. 363–373.

Spross, J., Cullen, M.L., et al. (Eds.). Update on nursing issues: Issues in chemotherapy administration. *Oncology Nursing Forum* 9(1), 1982, 50–54.

33. Amyloidosis

DEFINITION AND CAUSATIVE FACTORS

Amyloidosis is a condition that results from a proteinaceous, glassy, amorphous, extracellular substance infiltration into the skin, kidney, heart, GI tract, liver, lung, nerves, brain, bone marrow, joints, spleen, blood vessels, and eyes. It is classified as primary or secondary systemic or local deposition, hereditary, and age associated. Primary systemic amyloidosis is associated with multiple myeloma which usually results in cardiomyopathy (Chapter 16) and macroglossia (enlarged tongue). Secondary systemic amyloidosis is associated with Hodgkin disease and renal cell carcinoma causing nephropathy and renal failure. The cause of amyloidosis is unknown, but it is most probably a result of an absence of a proteolytic enzyme that breaks down the SAA protein, a serum protein that forms the amyloid AA protein. The liver seems to be responsible for synthesis of the amyloid AA protein which forms the amyloid substance. Amyloidosis is also thought to be related to IgG globulin (an immunoglobulin) misfunction. Multisystem involvement is possible with both primary and secondary forms. Amyloid deposition of the skin occurs from primary and secondary forms and local amyloidosis, and is characterized by raised, waxy, translucent papules, plaques, nodules, or tumefactions (swollen areas). With friction, these areas develop purpura. Amyloidosis involves all structures of the skin—epithelium, blood vessels, sweat and sebaceous glands, hair follicles, and subcutaneous tissues. the mucosa is also a target, and 50% of those with amyloidosis can be diagnosed by mucosal biopsy. Amyloidosis is a progressive, fatal disease, and the only treatment is supportive depending on the organ or systems involved. Death is usually caused by renal failure, heart failure, or arrhythmias.

Corresponding cancers include multiple myeloma, Hodgkin, kidney, hairy cell leukemia, thyroid, and all those treated with chemotherapy. Rheumatoid arthritis, tuberculosis, bronchiectasis, chronic osteomyelitis, connective tissue diseases, diabetes mellitus, myxedema, DIC, and inflammatory bowel diseases are additional causes.

ASSESSMENT DATA

- Raised waxy nodules on skin or mucosa
- Purpura
- Increased BUN and creatinine
- Oliguria or anuria
- Albuminuria
- Hepatosplenomegaly
- Carpal tunnel syndrome of wrist: Tinel sign
- Congestive heart failure
- Arrhythmias
- Hypoproteinemia
- Enlarged tongue
- Melena
- Peripheral neuropathy
- Hemoptysis
- Fibrinogenopenia
- Increased serum alkaline phosphatase
- Biopsy report positive for amyloidosis

NURSING DIAGNOSES

Impairment of skin integrity, related to skin and mucosal lesions and purpura, resulting from amyloid deposition.

Associated Nursing Diagnoses

1. Impaired urinary elimination, related to azotemia and renal cell cancer and amyloid deposition in the kidney (Chapter 35).

2. Altered cardiac output, decreased, related to an enlarged, flabby heart causing CHF, arrhythmias, and decreased tissue perfusion, resulting from amyloid deposition of the myocardium, endocardium, valves, and epicardium (Chapters 14 and 16).

3. Alteration in nutrition, deficit, related to infiltration of the tongue and GI tract mucosa by amyloid deposits causing obstruction, ulceration, malabsorption, hemorrhage, and protein loss (Chapters 12 and 38).

RATIONALE

Accumulation of proteinaceous substance within all structures of the skin causes impaired skin integrity.

Renal infiltrates of amyloid deposits impair urinary elimination. More critical with primary renal cell carcinoma.

Heart and blood vessel infiltration results in eventual decompensation of the heart muscle. More critical in the diagnosis of multiple myeloma.

Mechanical dysfunction as well as malabsorption compromise the host nutritionally.

4. Impaired physical mobility, related to amyloid deposition in bones and joints, causing osteoporosis and compression of median nerve (carpal tunnel syndrome).

Infiltration of bones, joints, and compression of nerves near joints reduces mobility mechanically and causes associated pain.

5. Sensory deficit, sight, related to amyloid deposits in any structure of the eye, causing impairment in eye acuity.

Increased proteinaceous substance in the eye results in blurring of vision.

6. Potential for physical injury, related to possible complications of amyloidosis—renal failure, decreased cardiac output, GI bleeding, decreased protein absorption, osteoporosis, decreased eye acuity, and decreased fibrinogen production causing bleeding.

Extradural deposits may produce compression of the brain, spinal cord, or cranial nerves potentiating physical injury.

7. Ineffective breathing pattern, related to diffuse involvement of bronchi and alveoli septa with amyloid deposition, causing hemoptysis and obstruction (Chapter 18).

Infiltration of the lung tissue and corresponding connective tissue causes inadequate pulmonary function.

NURSING INTERVENTIONS

Monitoring–Independent

1. Assess skin for lesions and record areas involved and type of lesion: papule, plaque, nodule, tumefactions (swelling); and purpura or bruises q 8 hr.
2. Assess oral cavity for presence of lesions and record location q 8 hr.
3. Assess all bony prominences for evidence of skin breakdown—redness, excoriations, blanching, and ulcer formation q 8 hr.
4. Accurate I and O and calculate I/O ratio for fluid balance q 8 and 24 hr.
5. Urine specific gravity q 8 hr.
6. Assess urine for protein qd.
7. Auscultate breath sounds in all lung fields and record changes q 8 hr.
8. Auscultate heart sounds in 4 valvular sites and record presence of gallop or murmur q 8 hr.
9. Assess client for dyspnea or orthopnea with each contact.

10. Assess client for difficulty swallowing, masticating, or speaking with each contact and prior to meals.

11. Auscultate bowel sounds in 4 quadrants and assess abdomen for rigidity and tenderness q 8 hr.

12. Hemocult all stools.

13. Assess peripheral motor status q 8 hr for ataxia and paresthesias, and wrist movement q 8 hr.

14. Assess LOC q 8 hr and record changes in awareness, orientation, and behavior.

15. BP, heart rate, respirations, temperature q 4 hr. BP and heart rate q 2 hr if cardiomyopathy suspected (route of temperature assessment depends on area of involvement).

16. Assess visual acuity using informal or formal methods of vision screening on admission, or when eye movement determined, qd.

17. Assess IV site for redness, swelling, and pain q 4 to 8 hr.

Monitoring–Interdependent

1. Assess laboratory data when available and compare to previous and normal values.

   Serum Alkaline Phosphatase: 13 to 39 IU (with liver involvement)
   BUN: 8 to 25 mg/dl
   Serum Creatinine: 0.6 to 1.5 mg/dl
   Serum Protein: 6.0 to 8.4 g/dl
   Serum Albumin: 3.5 to 5.0 g/dl
   Serum Fibrinogen: 0.15 to 0.35 g/dl
   Serum Calcium: 8.5 to 10.5 mg/dl
   Serum Phosphorus: 3.0 to 4.5 mg/dl
   Hemoglobin: 13 to 18 g/dl males
              12 to 16 g/dl females
   Hematocrit: 42 to 52% males
           37 to 48% females
   ABGs   pH: 7.35 to 7.45
          Po_2: 75 to 100 torr
          Pco_2: 35 to 45 torr
          HCO_3: 24 to 30 mEq/L
          BE: ± 2 mEq/L
          CO_2 Content: 24 to 30 mEq/L

2. Assess results of 12 lead EKG when available if cardiomyopathy expected—T wave changes, bundle branch block, P wave notching, or arrhythmias.

3. Assess results of chest x-ray if pulmonary or cardiac involvement occurs.

4. Assess results of barium enema when available if GI involvement occurs.

Change–Independent

1. Bathe without soap using commercially prepared bath emollients qd.
2. Eliminate all astringent solutions on affected skin areas including alcohol, lotions containing alcohol, powder, deodorant, and strong antiseptics.
3. Eliminate pressure on affected areas by using padding, eggcrate, or other device, for heel and elbow protection.
4. Offer fluids to 120 ml q hr alternating with milk and juice except if kidney or heart involvement has occurred.
5. Bedrest with minimized activity during acute phase of organ involvement.
6. O_2 at 2 L/min by nasal cannula if dyspnea or change in LOC due to hypoxia occurs.
7. Mouth care using a soft toothbruth and $\frac{1}{2}$ strength H_2O_2 pc and rinse thoroughly. Once a day, clean teeth with a mixture of H_2O_2 and baking soda to neutralize oral acid and remove plaque.
8. Turn, cough, deep breathe q 2 hr while on bedrest.
9. Active and passive ROME to all major joints q 4 hr while on bedrest if tolerated.
10. Lightly massage all unaffected bony prominences q 4 hr using non-astringent lotions.
11. Instruct client and/or family to request assistance when client desires to ambulate.
12. Assist client to perform ADLs while maintaining judicious independence and control over environment depending on physical limitations.
13. Eliminate all environmental hazards to safety. Keep side rails up and pad if client restless or disoriented. Keep bed in low position and place call light and personal articles within reach.
14. Explain condition and progress to client and family with each contact and assist them to ask questions and express concerns for the present and the future.
15. Include family members in plan of care and allow them to participate, if mutually therapeutic.

Change–Interdependent

1. Notify physician if:
    BUN greater than 30 mg/dl and creatinine greater than 2.0 mg/dl
    ABGs show uncompensated acidosis or Po_2 less than 75 mm Hg
    Serum protein less than 6.0 g/dl
    Serum albumin less than 3.5 g/dl
    BP systolic less than 90 mm Hg
    Gross rectal bleeding occurs

Hemoglobin less than 10 g/dl
Hematocrit less than 30%
Serum calcium less than 8 mg/dl
Arrhythmias occur

2. Consult with physician about diet high in protein and multivitamins (unless client in renal failure)

3. Consult with dietitian to assess client's food preferences and providing pureed foods in small frequent meals if macroglossia or malabsorption occurs. Hyperalimentation may be required with severe dysphagia.

4. Consult with respiratory therapist about possible benefits of incentive spirometry, IPPB, and other methods of maximizing pulmonary function and preventing complications if amyloidosis involves respiratory tract with recommendation to physician.

5. Consult with physical therapist about specific exercise routines appropriate to client's condition with bone or joint involvement and recommendation of physician.

6. D5W at KVO with cardiac, respiratory, or renal involvement or as prescribed by physician.

7. Anticipate physician to prescribe:
   Dialysis for severe renal failure
   Lasix to decrease fluid volume overload with CHF
   Digoxin to enhance cardiac contractility with CHF, cardiac myopathy
   Heparin to prevent thromboemboli
   Measures to correct hypocalcemia
   Multivitamins with GI tract involvement (other than obstruction)
   Antacids to decrease GI irritation
   Stool softener to decrease GI tract irritation
   Surgical correction of carpal tunnel syndrome
   Surgical removal of kidney tumor
   Frequent ABGs with respiratory involvement
   Blood coagulation studies to determine any impairment in addition to fibrinogenopenia (which can also occur with amyloidosis)

BIBLIOGRAPHY

Brodarick, S., Paine, R., Higa, E., and Carmichael, K.A. Pericardial tamponade: A new complication of amyloid heart disease. *The American Journal of Medicine,* **73,** 1982, 133–135.

Chapman, R.H., and Cotter, F. The carpal tunnel syndrome and amyloidosis. *Clinical Orthopaedics and Related Research,* **169,** 1982, 159–162.

Cohen, A.S. An update of clinical, pathologic, and biochemical aspects of amyloidosis. *International Journal of Dermatology,* **20**(8), 1981, 515–530.

Corbett, J.V. *Laboratory tests in nursing practice.* Norwalk, Connecticut: Appleton-Century-Crofts, 1982.

Gordon, M. *Manual of nursing diagnosis.* New York: McGraw-Hill, 1982.

Halter, S.K., DeLisa, J.A., Scardapane, D., and Sherrard, D.J. Carpal tunnel syndrome in chronic renal dialysis patients. *Arch Phys Med Rehabil,* **62**, 1981, 197–201.

Harvey, A.M., Johns, R.J., McKusick, V.A., Owens, A.H., Jr., and Ross, R.S. *The principles and practice of medicine* (20th ed.). New York: Appleton-Century-Crofts, 1980.

Keefer, C.S., and Wilkins, R.W. Median nerve syndromes. *Medicine, Essentials of Clinical Practice.* Boston: Little, Brown, 1970, pp. 991–992.

Levy, D.J., Franklin, G.O., and Rosenthal, W.S. Gastrointestinal bleeding and amyloidosis. *American Journal of Gastroenterology,* **77**(6), 1982, 422–426.

Linder, J., Silberman, H.R., and Croker, B.P. Amyloidosis complicating hairy cell leukemia. *American Journal of Clinical Pathologists,* **78**(6), 1982, 864–867.

Mead, M.G., Hickinbotham, P., and Walls, J. Amyloidosis localised to the bladder. *British Journal of Urology.* **54**(4), 1982, 428.

Miller, B.K. Carpal tunnel syndrome. *Nursing 80,* **10**(3), 1980, 50–53.

Pras, M., Franklin, E.C., Shibolet, S., and Frangione, B. Amyloidosis associated with renal cell carcinoma of the AA type. *The American Journal of Medicine,* **73**, 1982, 426–428.

34. Scalded Skin Syndrome

DEFINITION AND CAUSATIVE FACTORS

Scalded skin syndrome (SSS) is a group of conditions that have the appearance of skin scalded by hot water. The three most common conditions are staphylococcal-induced SSS, drug-induced SSS, and idiopathic SSS. Staphylococcal SSS is caused by strains of *Staphylococcus aureus* and produces skin eruptions in the immunosuppressed client with cancer. Clients with renal failure, visceral malignancy, or other debilitating conditions are also prone to staphylococcal SSS. It is manifested by a sudden onset of erythema and peeling of large areas of skin with underlying red, oozing, painful tissue. Healing occurs in 10 to 14 days without scarring.

Drug-induced SSS is thought to be a hypersensitivity drug reaction because many drugs appear to be associated with its occurrence. It is characterized by large areas of peeling skin and fever. Idiopathic SSS occurs primarily in the elderly, is recurrent, and is often fatal. SSS has a poor prognosis when it is concurrent with severe conditions, mortality being 50%, and there is no specific treatment. Infections, and fluid and electrolyte imbalances are potential complications.

Corresponding cancers include lymphoma and visceral malignancies. Sulfonamides, sulfones, pyrazolones, barbiturates, antibiotics, antiepileptic drugs, renal failure, and immunosuppression are additional causes.

A similar clinical picture may present in severe erythema multiforme or graft-versus-host disease.

ASSESSMENT DATA

- Widespread erythema
- Large areas of peeling skin
- Red, raw, and oozing under surface
- Pain
- Fever
- Stomatitis
- Fluid and electrolyte imbalances
- Conjunctival irritation

NURSING DIAGNOSES	RATIONALE
Alteration in skin integrity, related to large areas of peeling skin and raw, painful underlayers.	*Bacteria produce epidermolytic toxins, or adverse drug reactions cause toxic epidermal necrolysis.*

Associated Nursing Diagnoses

1. Fluid volume deficit related to oozing from large areas of skin surfaces.	Epidermal and dermal skin degradation results in large opened surface areas of skin.
2. Alteration in comfort level, related to painful skin lesions.	Inflammation and neuronal pain fiber stimulation.
3. Potential for infection related to possible infection and septicemia, resulting from exposed subcutaneous tissue.	Opened areas of skin and fluid environment are favorable for bacterial growth.

NURSING INTERVENTIONS

Monitoring–Independent

1. Assess all skin surfaces for onset, size and location of scaling, peeling, or exposed areas and record q 4 to 8 hr.
2. Oral temperature q 4 hr.
3. Inspect oral cavity for mucous membrane lesions q 8 hr.
4. Assess client for pain with each contact and record location, intensity, duration, and aggravating and alleviating factors.
5. Assess eyes for redness, itching, and swelling of eyelids q 8 hr.
6. Assess for painful or difficult swallowing with all po fluids.
7. Assess uninvolved areas for skin color, temperature, moisture, and turgor q 8 hr.
8. Accurate I and O and calculate I/O ratio for fluid balance q 8 and 24 hr.
9. Assess client for fatigue, weakness, and lethargy with each contact.
10. Assess LOC q 4 to 8 hr and record changes in awareness, orientation, and behavior.
11. Palpate peripheral pulses for bilateral quality and assess dependent areas for edema q 8 hr.
12. Auscultate breath sounds in all lung fields q 8 hr and record onset of cough and adventitious sounds.
13. BP, heart rate, and respirations q 4 hr.

14. Auscultate heart sounds in 4 valvular sites q 8 hr and record onset of gallop.
15. Auscultate bowel sounds in 4 quadrants q 8 hr and record onset of decreased, absent, or change in bowel sounds.

Monitoring–Interdependent

1. Assess laboratory data when available and compare to previous and normal values.

   Serum Sodium: 135 to 145 mEq/L
   Serum Potassium: 3.5 to 5.0 mEq/L
   Serum Chloride: 100 to 106 mEq/L
   Serum Calcium: 8.5 to 10.5 mg/dl
   BUN: 8 to 25 mg/dl
   Creatinine: 0.6 to 1.5 mg/dl
   Protein: total 6.0 to 8.4 g/dl
         albumin 3.5 to 5.0 g/dl
   CBC Hemoglobin: 13.0 to 18.0 g/dl males
                   12.0 to 16.0 g/dl females
         Hematocrit: 45 to 52% males
                   37 to 48% females
         RBC: 4.6 to $6.2 \times 10^6/mm^3$ males
            4.2 to $5.4 \times 10^6/mm^3$ females
         MCH: 27 to 32 pg
         MCHC: 32 to 36%
         MCV: 80 to 94 cu microns
         Platelets: 130,000 to 370,000 mm^3
         WBC: 4,500 to $11,500/mm^3$
   WBC Differential: Bands: 3%
                   Segs: 61%
                   Eosinophils: 4%
                   Basophils: 1%
                   Lymphocytes: 26%
                   Monocytes: 5%
   Culture and Sensitivity of Skin Lesions

2. Measure CVP if prescribed q 4 hr and compare to normal values: 4 to 8 mm H_2O.
3. Assess NG or Dobbhoff continuous feeding tube q 4 to 8 hr for correct placement or before each intermittent feeding (with severe stomatitis).
   Inject 10 ml air and auscultate gastric area for gurgle
   Aspirate for gastric contents and measure. If volume exceeds 100 ml, slow infusion rate or discontinue for 1 hr to prevent gastric distention and reflux aspiration, and auscultate bowel sounds to determine presence of peristalsis.

Change–Independent

1. Offer po fluids to 120 ml/hr while awake alternating with whole milk and juice.
2. Maintain bedrest with minimized activity with large areas of denuded skin and/or when fever present.
3. Turn, cough, deep breathe q 2 hr.
4. Bathe uninvolved areas cautiously using commercially prepared bath emollient or skin antiseptic, if prescribed.
5. Mouth care using soft toothbrush and $\frac{1}{2}$ strength H_2O_2 q 4 hr or after meals and rinse thoroughly. Once a day, clean teeth with a mixture of H_2O_2 and baking soda (except with stomatitis) to neutralize oral acid and remove plaque.
6. Massage all uninvolved bony areas with lotion q 4 hr.
7. Passive ROME to all major joints q 4 hr.
8. Institute all safety measures. Keep side rails up and pad if client restless or disoriented. Place call light and personal articles within reach, and ambulate with assistance.
9. Before all procedures, explain purpose and technique in understandable terms.
10. Assist client to perform ADLs and maintain judicious independence over self and environment within physical limitations.
11. Explain condition and progress to client and family with each contact. Assist them to ask questions and express concerns of the present and the future.
12. Include family members in plan of care and allow them to participate, if mutually beneficial.

Change–Interdependent

1. Notify physician if:
   WBC count greater than 11,500/mm^3
   Serum sodium less than 120 mEq/L or greater than 150 mEq/L
   Serum potassium less than 3.0 mEq/L or greater than 6.0 mEq/L
   Serum calcium less than 8.0 mg/dl or greater than 11.0 mg/dl
   Serum albumin less than 3.5 g/dl
   BUN greater than 30 mg/dl plus creatinine greater than 2.0 mg/dl
   Serum osmolality less than 280 mOsm/kg or greater than 300 mOsm/kg
   Onset of peeling skin
   CVP greater than 10 mm H_2O or less than 4 mm H_2O
   BP less than 90 torr systolic or greater than 160 torr
   Dysphagia occurs

2. Anticipate physician to prescribe:

NG or Dobbhoff feeding tube insertion with continuous or intermittent feedings if dysphagia occurs

Penicillinase-resistant antibiotics with potential onset of staphylococcal SSS or septicemia

Antibiotic eye ointment if conjunctivitis occurs

Corticosteroid therapy for drug-induced SSS and idiopathic SSS to minimize inflammatory response. Diet high in protein (contraindicated in renal failure), vitamins, fats, and carbohydrates

Oral pain medication

Potassium permanganate baths to prevent fungal infections

0.5% silver nitrate solution compresses to control bacterial growth and prevent water evaporation. Caution must be used with this solution because it can draw out sodium, potassium, magnesium, and calcium from the tissues. These compresses are soaked in silver nitrate solution, held in place with stretchy gauze (Kling), and changed q 3 to 4 hr.

Betadine solution soaks may be used as an alternative antimicrobial solution.

Corticosteroid creams applied in between soaks

Turning frame or net suspension bed as prescribed

3. Medicate appropriately for pain as prescribed and assess for effect in 20 to 30 min.

BIBLIOGRAPHY

Bergersen, B.S. *Pharmacology in nursing* (12th ed.). St. Louis: C.V. Mosby, 1973.

Corbett, J.V. *Laboratory tests in nursing practice.* Norwalk, Connecticut: Appleton-Century-Crofts, 1982.

Gordon, M. *Manual of nursing diagnosis.* New York: McGraw-Hill, 1982.

Luckman, J., and Sorensen, K.C. *Medical–surgical nursing—A psychophysiologic approach* (2nd ed.). Philadelphia: W.B. Saunders, 1980.

Safai, B. Life-threatening dermatologic complications of cancer. In A.D. Turnbull (Ed.), *Current problems in cancer* (Vol. 4, No. 4.). Chicago: Year Book Medical, 1979, pp. 5–8.

Sneddon, I.B., and Jackson, D. Emergencies in skin disease and burns. In C. Ogilvie (Ed.), *Birch's Emergencies in Medical Practice* (11th ed.). New York: Churchill Livingstone, 1981, Chap. 15.

PART VIII
ELIMINATION

---

35. Hyperuricemia

DEFINITION AND CAUSATIVE FACTORS

Hyperuricemia is an increase in the serum uric acid concentration from the normal range of 3.0 to 7.0 mg/dl. It is caused by a rapid destruction of cancer and healthy cells during radiation and chemotherapy (Table 35-1). Clients with acute and chronic myelogenous leukemia, acute lymphocytic leukemia, and myeloma have the greatest incidence. Uric acid levels can be as high as 20 mg/dl even before treatment is instituted. However, all clients undergoing rapid lysis of cancer cells are susceptible. Uric acid is an end product of purine (from nucleic acids) catabolism.

$$\text{Purines} \longrightarrow \text{Hypoxanthine} \xrightarrow[\text{Oxidase}]{\text{Xanthine}} \text{Xanthine} \xrightarrow[\text{Oxidase}]{\text{Xanthine}} \text{Uric acid}$$

Xanthines are water soluble but uric acid is not. Because uric acid is mainly excreted through the kidneys, it can precipitate in the distal tubule and collecting ducts of the nephron. Gouty nephropathy, uric acid nephrolithiasis, and acute hyperuricemic nephropathy are the possible end results, the latter causing renal obstruction, azotemia, and eventually renal failure. The classic diagnostic symptoms of hyperuricemic nephropathy are uric acid crystals in the urine and hyperuricemia. Allopurinol (a xanthine oxidase inhibitor), hydration, and alkalinizing the urine are the main prophylactic measures. Once kidney damage has occurred, it usually is irreversible. Hyperkalemia and hypocalcemia are often signs of kidney disease.

Corresponding cancers include acute and chronic myelogenous and acute lymphocytic leukemia, lymphoma, myeloma, and all cancers treated aggressively with chemotherapy or radiation. Dehydration, urine acidity, renal disease and obstruction uropathy are additional causes.

TABLE 35-1. CHEMOTHERAPEUTIC DRUGS THAT INCREASE URICEMIA

Busulfan (Myleran)	Mechlorethamine (Mustargen;
Carmustine (BCNU)	Nitrogen Mustard)
Chlorambucil (Leukeran)	Mercaptopurine (Purinethol)
Cyclophosphamide (Cytoxan)	Methotrexate
Hydroxyurea (Hydrea)	Thioguanine (Lanvis)

ASSESSMENT DATA

- Uric acid crystals in urine
- Serum uric acid greater than 7.0 mg/dl
- Elevated BUN and creatinine
- Hematuria
- Flank pain
- Nausea or vomiting
- Oliguria
- Acute renal failure
  Increased BUN and creatinine
  Decreased creatinine clearance
  Increased serum potassium
  Increased serum phosphorus
  Decreased serum calcium

Muscle twitching
Clotting defects, bleeding
Increased serum sodium
Hypertension
Weight gain
Edema
CHF, pulmonary edema
Anemia
Anorexia
Acidosis
Decreased serum proteins with proteinuria
Altered LOC, usually lethargy
Weakness and fatigue
Pruritis

NURSING DIAGNOSES

Altered urinary elimination pattern, decreased, related to the inability of the nephron to generate urine and eliminate waste.

Associated Nursing Diagnoses

1. Potential for physical injury, related to fluid volume overload, accumulation of waste products, and altered LOC.

2. Alteration in comfort level, related to acute flank pain, caused by renal calculi occluding the ureter.

RATIONALE

Lysis of cells and the buildup of uric acid in the collecting ducts of the nephrons inhibits elimination.

Hyperuricemia can precipitate progressive renal failure causing physical injury.

Build-up of uric acid crystals causes obstruction with neuronal stimulation manifesting the symptom of pain.

NURSING INTERVENTIONS

Monitoring–Independent

1. Hourly I and O and calculate I/O ratio for balance q 8 and 24 hr.
2. Assess urine for color and clarity q 1 hr.
3. Hemocult urine and obtain specific gravity q 8 hr.
4. Assess client for flank pain with each contact and record.
   Location
   Intensity
   Duration
   Radiation
   Aggravating and alleviating factors
5. Blood pressure, heart rate, and respirations q 2 to 4 hr.
6. Oral temperature q 4 hr.
7. Weigh q AM and compare to previous measurements (1 kg wt gain = 1000 ml approximate fluid retention provided caloric intake not excessive).
8. Auscultate breath sounds in all lung fields q 8 hr and record onset of adventitious sounds.
9. Auscultate heart sounds at 4 valvular sites q 8 hr and record changes in rate and onset of gallop.
10. Assess all dependent areas for edema q 8 hr.
11. Assess LOC q 8 hr and record changes in awareness, orientation, and behavior.
12. Assess cardiac monitor strip for changes in rhythm and onset of tall, peaked T waves (hyperkalemia) and prolonged ST segment (hypocalcemia) q 4 to 8 hr.
13. Assess skin color, temperature, and moisture q 8 hr.
14. Assess for tetany (hypocalcemia) with Chvostek and Trousseau signs. (Chvostek sign—positive if local spasm occurs following tapping of facial nerve; Trousseau sign—positive if muscle spasm occurs distally with application of tourniquet or BP cuff to upper arm.)
15. Assess objective and subjective indications of fatigue and weakness with each client contact.
16. Assess IV site for redness, pain, and swelling q 4 to 8 hr.

Monitoring–Interdependent

1. Assess laboratory data when available and compare to previous and normal values.
   Uric Acid: 3.0 to 7.0 mg/dl

BUN: 8 to 25 mg/dl
Serum Creatinine: 0.6 to 1.5 mg/dl
Serum Potassium: 3.5 to 5.0 mEq/L
Serum Chloride: 100 to 106 mEq/L
Serum Calcium: 8.5 to 10.5 mg/dl
Serum Phosphorus: 3.0 to 4.5 mg/dl
Serum Sodium: 135 to 145 mEq/L
Urine pH: 4.5 to 8.0
Creatinine Clearance: 100 to 120 ml/min
Urine for uric acid crystals
Urinalysis positive for blood, WBC, protein
Hemoglobin: 12 to 16 g/dl females
            14 to 18 g/dl males
Hematocrit: 37 to 48% females
          45 to 52% males
ABGs   pH: 7.35 to 7.45
        Po_2: 75 to 100 torr
        Pco_2: 35 to 45 torr
        HCO_3: 24 to 30 mEq/L
        BE: ± 2 mEq/L
        CO_2 Content: 24 to 30 mEq/L

2. Assess for side effects of allopurinol (Zyloprim).

Skin rash, nausea and/or vomiting, diarrhea (most common), fever, sore throat, malaise, anemia, leukopenia, thrombocytopenia, headache, dizziness, nephritis, or hepatomegaly.

Change–Independent

1. Bedrest with active and passive ROME to all major joints q 6 hr with onset of symptoms.

2. Turn, cough, deep breathe q 2 hr.

3. Apply ice collar to neck with onset of nausea.

4. Bathe daily, without soap, using commercially prepared bath emollient qd.

5. Back care using nonastringent lotions to all bony areas q 4 hr, except areas of radiation.

6. Mouth care using soft toothbrush and mouthwash q 4 hr. Once a day, clean teeth with a mixture of H_2O_2 and baking soda to neutralize oral acid and remove plaque.

7. Offer fluids to 120 ml q 1 hr alternating with fat free milk and non-citrus juice (both low in purines) *IF* no kidney damage demonstrable (fluids high in volume, potassium, and protein would be limited).

8. Explain condition and progress to client and family with each contact. Assist them to ask questions and express concerns of the present and the future.

9. Include family members in plan of care and allow them to participate, if mutually therapeutic.

10. Institute all safety measures and pad side rails if client restless or disoriented.

11. Assist client to perform ADLs and maintain judicious independence and control over self and environment within physical limitations.

Change–Interdependent

1. D5W at KVO or as prescribed by physician.

2. Medicate appropriately for pain as prescribed and assess effects in 10 to 20 min.

3. Notify physician if:
   Serum uric acid greater than 7.0 mg/dl
   Urinary output less than 30 ml/hr
   Hematuria occurs with or without flank pain
   Weight gain exceeds 1 kg/day with elevation in blood pressure, lung congestion, or edema
   BUN greater than 25 mg/dl and creatinine greater than 1.5 mg/dl
   Serum calcium less than 8.5 mg/dl
   Serum potassium greater than 6.0 mEq/L
   Blood pH less than 7.30
   Hemoglobin less than 10 g/dl
   Hematocrit less than 30%

4. Anticipate physician to prescribe:
   Prior to chemotherapy or radiation
   Allopurinol 300 to 600 mg to prevent elevations in serum uric acid
   IV fluids of 3000 ml/day to rigorously hydrate client
   $NaHCO_3$ 6 to 8 g/day IV or 3 g po to alkalinize urine to 7.0 to 7.5
   With renal failure
   Mannitol IV to stimulate diuresis
   If unsuccessful and uric acid levels 25 to 30 mg/dl, dialysis will be required.
   Fluid restriction to minimize hypervolemia
   Aldomet to decrease blood pressure
   IV glucose with insulin or Kayexalate po or enema to reduce serum potassium levels
   IV push $NaHCO_3$ if acidosis severe
   Diet with restricted protein, potassium, and salt. Usually 20 to 40 g

protein, 500 mg sodium and potassium but varies according to degree of failure

Frequent laboratory work to monitor BUN and creatinine

BIBLIOGRAPHY

Brundage, D.J. *Nursing management of renal problems* (2nd ed.). St. Louis: C.V. Mosby, 1980.

Corbett, J.V. *Laboratory tests in nursing practice*. Norwalk, Connecticut: Appleton-Century-Crofts, 1982.

DeVita, V.T., Hellman, S., and Rosenburg, S.A. *Cancer, principles, and practice of oncology*. Philadelphia: J.B. Lippincott, 1982.

Gordon, M. *Manual of nursing diagnosis*. New York: McGraw-Hill, 1982.

Giovoni, L.E., and Hayes, J.E. *Drugs and nursing implications* (4th ed.). Norwalk, Connecticut: Appleton-Century-Crofts, 1982.

Hull, A.R. Complications of uremia. *Urologic Clinics of North America*, 9(2), 1982, 275–278.

Johanson, B.C., Dungca, C., Hoffmeister, D., et al.   *Standards for critical care.* St. Louis: C.V. Mosby, 1981.

Knochel, J.P. The pathophysiology of uremia. *Hospital Practice*, 16(12), 1981, 65-76.

Marino, L.B. *Cancer nursing*. St. Louis: C.V. Mosby, 1981.

See-Lasley, K., and Ignoffo, R.J. *Manual of oncology therapeutics*. St. Louis: C.V. Mosby, 1981.

36. Obstructive Uropathy

Obstructive uropathy is a condition that results from a neoplasm of the kidney, ureter, or urethra, or from direct extension of a malignancy in adjacent structures causing obstruction of the urinary flow. The incidence of renal cell carcinoma is 1 to 2% of all cancers; ureteral and urethral neoplasms can occur, but they are rare. Bladder cancers usually do not cause obstruction unless the tumor is extremely large and far advanced, or the bladder becomes fibrotic and contracted from radiochemotherapy. Ureteral obstruction is most frequently caused by cancer of the cervix, and it can result in urinary stasis, infection, renal calculi, and eventually, hydronephrotic atrophy of the kidney with destruction of the nephrons. The incidence of bilateral ureteral involvement is 33.3% to 50%. Renal insufficiency, renal failure, and uremia, characterized by an increase in BUN, creatinine, serum potassium, and circulating blood volume, are the end results. Flank pain, oliguria and/or anuria, and a palpable abdominal mass are distinguishing manifestations. Urethral obstruction is most commonly caused by prostate cancer resulting in backflow to the bladder and distention.

Corresponding cancers include cervix, prostate, kidney, ovary, bladder, colon, retroperitoneal tumors, lymphoma, sarcomas, multiple myeloma, pancreas, and breast. Renal calculi, strictures, periurethral fibrosis, blood clots, high dose abdominal radiation, aortic aneurysms, and neuromuscular dysfunction are additional causes.

ASSESSMENT DATA

- Ureteral obstruction
  Urinary retention
  Hematuria
  Acute flank pain
  Pyemia

Fever, chills
Palpable abdominal mass
- Acute renal failure
  Increased BUN and serum creatinine
  Edema, weight gain, hypertension
  Increased serum potassium, sodium, chloride
  Metabolic acidosis
  Decreased creatinine clearance
- Bladder obstruction
  Hematuria—usually bright red with clots
  Urgency sensations
- Urethral obstruction
  Decreased urinary stream
  Urinary frequency, urgency
  Bladder fullness and pressure sensations
- X-ray determination of obstruction (urocystogram, excretory urogram, retrograde pyelogram, radioisotope renogram)

NURSING DIAGNOSES

Altered urinary elimination pattern, decreased, related to obstruction of urine flow from the kidney, resulting in urinary retention, renal destruction, and failure.

Associated Nursing Diagnoses

1. Impaired urinary elimination, retention, related to inability of urine to flow from the bladder.

2. Alteration in comfort level, related to obstruction that causes acute or colicky flank pain, and fever.

RATIONALE

Primary cancers of the urinary system and invasive cancers cause renal obstruction due to tumor load. Most common is Wilms tumor and invasion from lymphomas and multiple myeloma.

Primary cancers of the urinary system (bladder, urethral neck) and invasive cancers (prostate, cervix, ovary, pancreas) cause urinary obstruction due to tumor load.

Neuronal stimulation is enhanced by a full bladder leading to pain. Stasis of urine in the bladder lends itself to growth of bacteria causing a rise in temperature.

NURSING INTERVENTIONS

Monitoring–Independent

1. Hourly I and O and calculate I/O ratio for fluid balance q 8 and 24 hr.

2. Assess urine for color and clarity q 1 hr.

3. Assess for bladder distention by palpation, percussion, or measurement according to predetermined reference points (umbilicus) q 8 hr.

4. Hemocult urine and determine specific gravity q 8 hr.

5. Assess client for pain with each contact and record.
   Location
   Intensity
   Duration
   Radiation
   Aggravating and alleviating factors

6. BP, heart rate, and respirations q 2 to 4 hr.

7. Oral temperature q 4 hr.

8. Weigh q AM and compare to previous measurements.

9. Auscultate breath sounds in all lung fields q 8 hr and record onset of rales, rhonchi, and wheeze.

10. Auscultate heart sounds at 4 valvular sites q 8 hr and record changes in rate or onset of gallop.

11. Inspect ankles and sacrum for edema q 8 hr.

12. Palpate peripheral pulses for bilateral quality q 8 hr.

13. Assess LOC q 4 to 8 hr and record changes in awareness, orientation, and behavior.

14. Assess cardiac monitor strip for changes in rhythm and onset of tall peaked T waves (hyperkalemia) and prolonged ST segment (hypocalcemia) q 4 to 8 hr.

15. Assess skin color, temperature, and moisture q 8 hr.

16. Assess for tetany (hypocalcemia) with Chvostek and Trousseau signs. (Chvostek—positive, if local spasm occurs following tapping of facial nerve; Trousseau sign—positive if muscle spasm occurs distally with application of tourniquet to upper arm.)

17. Assess objective and subjective indications of fatigue and weakness with each client contact.

18. Assess IV site for redness, pain, and swelling q 4 to 8 hr.

Monitoring–Interdependent

1. Assess laboratory data when available and compare to previous and normal values.

	NORMAL	RENAL FAILURE
BUN	8–25 mg/dl	Increased
Serum Creatinine	0.6–1.5 mg/dl	Increased
Creatinine Clearance	100–120 ml/min	Decreased
Serum Potassium	3.5–5.0 mEq/L	Increased
Serum Sodium	135–145 mEq/L	Increased
Serum Calcium	8.5–10.5 mg/100 ml	Decreased
Serum Chloride	100–106 mEq/L	Increased
Serum Phosphorus	3.0–4.5 mg/dl	Increased

> *Urinalysis:* positive for blood, WBC, protein
> *Hemoglobin:* 12 to 16 g/dl females
>   14 to 18 g/dl males
> *Hematocrit:* 37 to 48% females
>   45 to 52% males
> *ABGs*   pH: 7.35 to 7.45
> Po_2: 75 to 100 torr
> Pco_2: 35 to 45 torr
> HCO_3: 24 to 30 mEq/L
>   BE: ± 2 mEq/L
> CO_2 Content: 24 to 30 mEq/L
> *WBCs:* 4,500 to 11,500/mm^3

2. Assess functioning of cystostomy, nephrostomy, pyelostomy, cutaneous ureterostomy, or ureterostomy in situ (used to relieve acute urinary obstruction until a permanent urinary diversion is performed surgically) q 1 hr noting amount, color, and character of drainage (Fig. 36-1).

3. Assess insertion site of catheter for redness and swelling with each dressing change. (Maintain strict sterility of insertion site; it is a direct pathway of organisms to the kidney with serious risk of infection.)

Change–Independent

1. Bedrest with minimized activity with onset of symptoms.
2. Turn, cough, and deep breathe q 2 hr.
3. Bathe, without soap, using commerically prepared bath emollient qd.
4. Back care using nonastringent lotions with friction massage to all bony areas q 4 hr.
5. Mouth care with antiseptic oral agents and soft toothbrush q 4 hr. Once a day, clean teeth with a mixture of H_2O_2 and baking soda to neutralize oral acid and remove plaque.

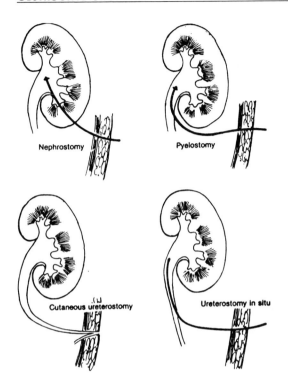

Nephrostomy

Pyelostomy

Cutaneous ureterostomy

Ureterostomy in situ

Figure 36-1. Methods of supravesicular urinary diversions for relieving the obstruction of the upper urinary tract. Source: DeVita, et al., 1982, with permission.

6. Offer fluids to 120 ml q hr after insertion of nephrostomy, ureterostomy, cystostomy, or Foley catheter *IF* no kidney damage or renal failure demonstrable.

7. Institute all safety measures in environment and pad side rails if client restless or disoriented.

8. Active and passive ROME to all major joints while on bedrest q 4 to 8 hr.

9. Assist client to perform ADLs and maintain judicious independence and control over self and environment within physical limitations.

10. Explain condition and progress to client and family with each contact. Assist them to ask questions and express concerns of the present and the future.

11. Include family members in plan of care and allow them to participate, if mutually therapeutic.

Change–Interdependent

1. D5W at KVO or as prescribed by physician.

2. Medicate appropriately for pain or fever as prescribed and assess effect in 10 to 20 min.

3. Notify physician if:
    Urinary output less than 30 ml/hr
    Hematuria occurs in combination with acute flank pain
    Temperature elevates to 101.0°F or greater
    Weight gain exceeds 1 kg/day with elevation in blood pressure, lung
        congestion, or edema
    BUN greater than 25 mg/dl and creatinine greater than 1.5 mg/dl
    Serum potassium greater than 6.0 mEq/L
    Blood pH less than 7.30
    Hemoglobin less than 10 g/dl
    Serum calcium less than 8.5 mg/dl
    Hematocrit less than 30%
4. Anticipate the physician to prescribe:
    Foley catheter insertion for urethral obstruction
    Antibiotics to eliminate or prevent infection (those *not* nephrotoxic)
    With renal failure
        Dialysis to normalize blood chemistries and fluid balance
        Fluid restriction to minimize hypervolemia
        Aldomet to decrease blood pressure
        IV glucose with insulin or Kayexalate po or by enema to reduce serum
            potassium levels
        Amphogel to combine with phosphorus in the GI tract and then
            eliminated (calcium is decreased in renal failure and phosphorus is
            increased because of their inversely proportional relationship and
            regulation)
        IV push $NaHCO_3$ if acidosis severe
        Diet with restricted protein, potassium, and salt. Usually 20 to 40 g
            protein, 500 mg sodium and potassium but varies according to de-
            gree of failure.
        Frequent laboratory work to monitor BUN and creatinine
    Allopurinol 200 mg po TID
    Ultrasound of the abdomen
    Temporary nephrostomy

BIBLIOGRAPHY

Abbeloff, M.D., and Lenhand, R. Clinical management of urethral obstruction sec-
    ondary to malignant lymphoma. *Johns Hopkins Medical Journal*, **134**, 1974, 34–36.
Barrett, N. Cancer of the bladder—A case history. *American Journal of Nursing*,
    81(12), 1981, 2192–2195.
Corbett, J.V. *Laboratory tests in nursing practice*. Norwalk, Connecticut: Appleton-
    Century-Crofts, 1982.

DeVita, V.T., Hellman, S., and Rosenburg, S.A. Acute obstructive uropathy. In V.T. DeVita, et al. (Eds.), *Cancer, principles and practice of oncology*. Philadelphia: J.B. Lippincott, 1982, pp. 1618–1621.

Gordon, M. *Manual of nursing diagnosis*. New York: McGraw-Hill, 1982.

Grabstald, H. Urinary tract emergencies in the cancer patient. In A.D. Turnbull (Ed.) *Current problems in cancer* (Vol. 4, No. 4,). Chicago: Year Book Medical, 1979, pp. 27–29.

Portlock, C.S., and Gaffinet, D.R. *Manual of clinical problems in oncology*. Boston: Little, Brown, 1980.

Sise, J.G., and Crichlow, R.W. Obstruction due to malignant tumors. In J. Yarbro and R. Bornstein (Eds.), *Oncologic emergencies*. New York: Grune and Stratton, 1981, pp. 97–118.

Taylor, P.T. Untreated cervical cancer complicated by obstructive uropathy. *Gynecologic Cancer*, 2, 1981, 167.

Townsend, C.E. Obstructive uropathy relevant to the client with cancer. Paper presented at the *First Oncology Nursing Seminar, Clemson University*, College of Nursing, Clemson, South Carolina, May 1980.

PART IX
NUTRITION

37. Small Bowel Obstruction

DEFINITION AND CAUSATIVE FACTORS

Small bowel obstruction in the client with cancer occurs because of either a primary malignancy of the GI tract or of metastasis of the GI tract. Carcinoid tumors, those which spread through mucosal tracts, commonly cause obstruction as these cells invade a section of the bowel resulting in fibrosis and contraction of tissue. Encirclement of the bowel by the tumor causes lumen narrowing and partial obstruction, but eventually complete obstruction will result. Metastatic tumors are the most frequent cause of obstruction: colorectum (44.8%), ovary (16.8%), and cervix (14.6%). Perforation of the obstructed area is a rare sequela. Physical indications in the client will depend on location in the GI tract and degree of obstruction, partial or complete (Table 37-1). Intestinal obstruction is treated conservatively initially; surgical intervention is performed only when conservative measures fail or if the obstruction is complete.

Corresponding cancers include primary small bowel—carcinoid, adenocarcinoma, sarcoma, lymphoma, and melanoma (1 to 3%)—and metastatic colorectal, ovary, cervix, pancreas, and gastric. Radiation necrosis and chronic constipation are additional causes.

ASSESSMENT DATA

- Abdominal pain
- Abdominal distention
- Nausea and vomiting
- High pitched, hyperactive bowel sounds proximal to obstruction

- Diminished or absent bowel sounds distal to obstruction
- Constipation
- Oliguria
- Dehydration

243

TABLE 37-1. DIFFERENTIATING OBSTRUCTION
OF THE SMALL INTESTINE

Signs	High Small Intestine	Low Small Intestine	Partial	Complete
Pain	Intense	Present but intensity varies	Crampy	Constant
Distention	Present but not severe	Present and severe	Present	Abdomen turgid and greatly enlarged
Vomiting	Severe	Present and may contain fecal material	Present but degree varies	Severe
Abnormal bowel sounds	Diminished or absent	High pitched, frequent proximal to obstruction, diminished or absent distally	Same	Same but will be absent distally
Oliguria (late sign)	Present	Usually does not occur unless vomiting severe	Varies	Varies, present with onset of shock

NURSING DIAGNOSES

Alteration in nutrition, less than body requirements, related to the inability of food to transgress through the digestive process, because of mechanical obstruction of the bowel.

Associated Nursing Diagnoses

1. Potential fluid volume deficit, related to loss of fluid and electrolytes through vomiting, and/or NG tube suction.
2. Alterations in comfort level, acute pain, related to retention

RATIONALE

Primary functions of the small intestine are digestion of carbohydrates, fats, and proteins and absorption of the end products of digestion. This process is impaired with intestinal obstruction.

The stomach acts as a reservoir for food and begins to digest proteins.

Increased lumen pressure leads to an increase in capillary perme-

of fluid, edema, and intestinal wall necrosis, resulting from increased pressure on the lumen of the small bowel.

ability and extravasation of fluid and electrolytes into the peritoneal cavity.

NURSING INTERVENTIONS

Monitoring–Independent

1. Auscultate bowel sounds in 4 quadrants q 2 to 4 hr and record changes in pitch and frequency of sound.
2. Assess client for abdominal pain with each contact and describe.
   Location
   Radiation
   Intensity
   Associated symptoms: nausea, vomiting, diaphoresis, increased BP, and heart rate
   Aggravating and alleviating factors
3. Palpate abdomen for rebound, general tenderness, and firmness q 2 to 4 hr.
4. Measure abdominal girth using umbilicus as reference point q 8 hr.
5. Assess presence or absence of flatus and stools q 8 hr.
6. Hourly I and O and calculate I/O ratio for fluid balance q 8 hr and 24 hr. Specify vomitus amount.
7. Urine specific gravity q 8 hr.
8. Oral temperature q 4 hr.
9. Weigh q AM before breakfast and compare to previous measurement.
10. BP, heart rate, and respirations q 2 hr with onset of symptoms.
11. Assess LOC q 8 hr and record changes in awareness, orientation, and behavior.
12. Assess client for hyperosmotic dehydration q 4 to 8 hr.
    Poor muscle turgor
    Tachycardia
    Dry mucous membranes
    Dry, hot skin
    Oliguria
    Hypotension
13. Assess client for hypokalemia q 8 hr.
    Flat T wave and U wave on cardiac monitor
    Arrhythmias

Fatigue, weakness, lethargy
Irritability, confusion

Monitoring–Interdependent

1. Assess for gastric placement of NG tube by injecting 10 to 20 ml of air and ascultating for gastric gurgle q 4 to 8 hr.
2. Assess amount and character of gastric secretions removed by NG or Miller–Abbott tube q 4 to 8 hr.
3. Hemocult vomitus and/or NG tube secretions q 6 hr.
4. Assess results of laboratory data when available and compare to previous and normal values.
   Serum Sodium: 135 to 145 mEq/L
   Serum Potassium: 3.5 to 5.0 mEq/L
   Serum Chloride: 100 to 106 mEq/L
   Serum Calcium: 8.5 to 10.5 mg/dl
   Serum Magnesium: 1.5 to 2.0 mEq/L
   Serum Phosphate: 3.0 to 4.5 mg/dl
   Serum Osmolality: 286 to 294 mOsm/kg
   Serum Proteins: 6.0 to 8.0 g/dl
   Serum Albumin: 3.5 to 5.5 g/dl
   BUN: 8 to 25 mg/dl
   Creatinine: 0.6 to 1.5 mg/dl
   Blood Sugar: 70 to 100 mg/dl
   CBC: Hemoglobin: 13.0 to 18.0 g/dl males
                        12.0 to 16.0 g/dl females
             Hematocrit: 45 to 52% males
                         37 to 48% females
             RBC: 4.6 to 6.2×10^6/mm^3 males
                   4.2 to 5.4×10^6/mm^3 females
             MCH: 27 to 32 pg
             MCHC: 32 to 36%
             MCV: 80 to 94 cu microns
             Platelets: 130,000 to 370,000 mm^3
5. Urine sugar and acetone q 6 hr if TPN prescribed and solution contains more than 5% glucose.

Change–Independent

1. Maintain bedrest with minimized activity.
2. Irrigate NG tube with 20 ml of saline q 4 hr.
3. Bathe, without soap, using commercially prepared bath emollient daily.

4. Apply ice collar to neck with onset of nausea.
5. Provide cool environment if applicable.
6. Mouth care q 6 hr using $\frac{1}{2}$ strength H_2O_2 and soft toothbrush, or after each vomiting episode. Once a day, clean teeth with a mixture of H_2O_2 and baking soda to neutralize oral acid and remove plaque.
7. Back care q 4 hr with deep massage to all bony prominences with nonastringent lotion.
8. Turn, cough, and deep breathe q 2 hr.
9. Passive ROME to all major joints q 6 hr.
10. Maintain frequent physical and visual contact with client during acute phase stating time of return before leaving.
11. Institute all safety measures by elevating side rails and pad if client is restless, placing bed in low position, and arranging call light and personal articles within easy reach.
12. Explain condition and progress to client and family with each contact. Assist them to ask questions and express concerns of the present and the future.
13. Include family members in plan of care and allow them to participate, if mutually therapeutic.

Change–Interdependent

1. Medicate appropriately for pain as prescribed and assess effect in 10 to 20 min.
2. Notify physician if:
   Bowel sounds change to high pitch with hyperactivity and identify quadrants
   Bowel sounds change to diminished or absent and identify quadrants
   Acute onset of vomiting
   Acute onset of abdominal pain occurs and abdomen becomes distended (increased abdominal girth)
   Hematocrit less than 30%
   Blood sugar less than 60 mg/dl or greater than 350 mg/dl
   WBC greater than 12,000/mm^3
   Hemoglobin less than 10 g/dl
   Urine S and A greater than +1 and trace (with TPN)
   Serum sodium less than 135 mEq/L or greater than 145 mEq/L
   Serum potassium less than 3.0 mEq/L or greater than 5.0 mEq/L
   pH greater than 7.5
   Urinary output less than 30 ml/hr or greater than 200 ml/hr (may indicate overhydration with IV fluids)

3. Anticipate physician to prescribe:
   Nasogastric or Miller–Abbot tube insertion
   NPO
   IV electrolyte solutions
   Potassium to IV with serum potassium less than 3.2 mEq/L
   Barium enema
   TPN if NPO greater than 3 days
   Surgical intervention if conservative therapy unsuccessful
   Rectal aspirin/acetaminophen suppositories for elevated temperature

BIBLIOGRAPHY

Corbett, J.V. *Laboratory tests in nursing practice*. Norwalk, Connecticut: Appleton-Century-Crofts, 1982.

Gordon, M. *Manual of nursing diagnosis*. New York: McGraw-Hill, 1982.

Harvey, A.M., Johns, R.J., McKusick, V.A., Owens, A.H., and Ross, R.S. *The principles and practice of medicine* (20th ed.) New York: Appleton-Century-Crofts, 1980.

Horton, J., and Hill, G.J. *Clinical oncology*. Philadelphia: W.B. Saunders, 1977.

Kinney, M.R., et al. *A.A.C.N.'s clinical reference for critical care nursing*. New York: McGraw-Hill, 1981.

Luckman, J., and Sorensen, K.C. *Medical–surgical nursing—A psychophysiologic approach* (2nd ed.). Philadelphia: W.B. Saunders, 1980.

Patras, A.Z. The operation's over, but the danger's not. *Nursing 82*, 12(9), 1982, 50–56.

Sise, J.G., and Crichlow, R.W. Obstruction due to malignant tumors. J. Yarbro and R. Bornstein (Eds.), *Oncologic emergencies*. New York: Grune and Stratton, 1981, pp. 97–118.

Wilson, R.E. Surgical emergencies—Obstructive disease. In V.T. DeVita, S. Hellman, S.A. Rosenberg (Eds.), *Cancer, principles and practice in oncology*. Philadelphia: J.B. Lippincott, 1982.

38. Malabsorption Syndrome

DEFINITION AND CAUSATIVE FACTORS

Malabsorption syndrome develops to some degree in the client who has cancer in any structure of the GI tract. Although fat malabsorption is most commonly associated with this syndrome, other nutrients are also involved depending on the site of the malignant growth. Cancer of the stomach produces a deficiency of the intrinsic factor necessary for vitamin B_{12} absorption. Pancreatic cancer decreases the production of fat and protein enzymes, and lymphomas cause lymphatic obstruction preventing the absorption of fats via the lymphatics. Cancers of the esophagus, stomach, and colon produce a condition known as enteropathy, inflammation and ulceration of the GI tract, preventing protein absorption. Fat soluble vitamins (A, E, D, K), folic acid, B vitamins, iron, and electrolyte (sodium, potassium, phosphorus, chloride, calcium, magnesium) deficiencies also occur.

Corresponding cancers include gastric, gallbladder, pancreas, small and large intestines, and metastatic tumors that invade the GI tract. Gastrectomy, bowel resection, intestinal obstruction, high dose chemotherapy, and intestinal radiation are additional causes.

ASSESSMENT DATA

- Steatorrhea
- Increased appetite accompanied with weight loss
- Abdominal distention
- Foul smelling diarrhea
- Silver gray or yellow stools
- Anemia (iron deficiency)
- Parasthesies (vitamin B complex deficiency)
- Bleeding, bruising (vitamin K deficiency)
- Tetany (calcium deficiency)
- Pathologic fractures (vitamin D deficiency)

- Edema (protein deficiency)
- Skin and vision changes (vitamin A deficiency)
- Dehydration
- Decreased serum electrolytes

NURSING DIAGNOSES	RATIONALE
Alteration in nutrition, less than body requirements, related to inability of the GI tract to absorb nutrients, resulting in malnutrition.	*Impaired intestinal mucosal absorption of carbohydrates, fats, proteins, electrolytes, and/or vitamins.*

Associated Nursing Diagnoses

1. Altered cardiac output, decreased, related to potential bleeding and anemia that results from a deficiency of vitamin K, iron, and protein.

Vitamin K is synthesized by bacteria in the large intestine and is essential for prothrombin formation. Iron is essential for transporting oxygen to tissues. Protein enzymes are necessary for fat transport as energy source.

2. Potential for physial injury, related to vitamins B_{12} and D, and calcium deficiencies, resulting in possible pathologic fractures or tetany.

Vitamin B_{12} deficiency causes neurologic abnormalities as a result of patchy degeneration of the central and peripheral nervous systems. Vitamin D assists in the absorption of calcium which is necessary for bone formation and maintenance as well as neuromuscular activity.

3. Sensory deficit, uncompensated, related to decreases in visual acuity and tactile sensation, resulting from vitamin A and B_{12} deficiencies.

Vitamin A is essential for visual adaptation to light and dark. Vitamin B_{12} is essential for nervous system function.

NURSING INTERVENTIONS

Monitoring–Independent

1. Assess bowel sounds in all 4 quadrants for pitch and frequency of sounds q 2 to 4 hr and record changes.

2. Record number, color, odor, and amount of all stools. Hemocult all stools.
3. Weigh q A.M. before breakfast and compare to previous measurements.
4. Measure abdominal girth using predetermined reference points qd.
5. Assess dependent areas for edema and measure ankles using premarked reference points qd.
6. BP, heart rate, and respirations q 4 to 8 hr.
7. Assess client for degree of fatigue and weakness q 8 hr using objective and subjective criteria.
8. Assess skin for turgor, bruises, muscle mass, and dryness qd.
9. Assess client for pain in abdomen, joints, and long bones q 8 hr.
10. Assess for positive Trousseau sign by inflating blood pressure cuff for 1 to 5 min inducing carpal spasm and positive Chvostek sign by tapping the facial nerve just below the temple inducing contraction of the lip, nose, face q 8 hr indicating tetany (hypocalcemia).
11. Accurate I and O and calculate I/O ratio for fluid balance q 8 and 24 hr.
12. Temperature q 4 hr.
13. Assess LOC q 8 hr and record changes in awareness, orientation, and behavior.
14. Auscultate heart sounds in 4 valvular sites q 8 hr and record onset of extra heart sounds.
15. Auscultate breath sounds in all lung fields q 8 hr and record onset of adventitious sounds.

Monitoring–Interdependent

1. Assess results of laboratory data when available and compare to previous and normal values.
   Schilling Test: greater than 7%
   Serum vitamin B_{12}: 90 to 280 pg/ml
   Serum Folic Acid: greater than 1.9 ng/dl
   Total Protein: 6.0 to 8.0 g/dl
   Albumin: 3.5 to 5.5 g/dl
   CBC   Hemoglobin: 13.0 to 18.0 g/dl males
                    12.0 to 16.0 g/dl females
         Hematocrit: 45 to 52% males
                    37 to 48% females
         RBC: 4.6 to 6.2 × 10⁶/mm³ males
              4.2 to 5.4 × 10⁶/mm³ females
         MCH: 27 to 32 pg.
         MCHC: 32 to 36%
         MCV: 80 to 94 cu microns

Platelets: 130,000 to 370,000 mm³
WBC: 4,500 to 11,500/mm³
Prothrombin Time: control + 4 sec
Partial Thromboplastin Time: Control + 10 sec
Blood Sugar: 70 to 100 mg/dl
Serum Sodium: 135 to 145 mEq/L
Serum Potassium: 3.5 to 5.0 mEq/L
Serum Chloride: 100 to 106 mEq/L
Serum Calcium: 8.5 to 10.5 mg/dl
Serum Cholesterol: 140 to 330 mg/dl
Serum Magnesium: 1.5 to 2.0 mEq/L
Serum Phosphorus: 3.0 to 4.5 mg/dl
Serum Amylase: 4 to 25 U/ml
Stool Fat: less than 7 g/24 hr

2. Assess urine for sugar and acetone q 6 hr if TPN prescribed and solution contains more than 5% dextrose (Chapter 39).

3. Assess IV site or central line insertion site for pain, redness, or swelling q 8 hr.

Change–Independent

1. Maintain bedrest with minimized activity and assisted ambulation.
2. Offer fluids to 120 ml q hr alternating with fat free milk and juice of choice or as tolerated.
3. Back care q 4 hr while on bedrest with massage to all bony prominences.
4. Mouth care after meals using soft toothbrush with $\frac{1}{2}$ strength H_2O_2 and rinse thoroughly. Once a day, clean teeth with a mixture of H_2O_2 and baking soda to neutralize oral acid and remove plaque.
5. Bathe with commercially prepared emollient instead of soap.
6. Passive ROME to all major joints 3 times q 4 hr while on bedrest.
7. Apply O_2 at 2 L/min by nasal cannula with onset of SOB of dyspnea on exertion.
8. File fingernails to shortest length and soft brush clean every day.
9. Cleanse rectal area after each diarrheal stool and apply protective agent.
10. Turn, cough, deep breathe q 2 hr while on bedrest.
11. Progress activity gradually each day with assistance according to tolerance.
12. Assist client to perform ADLs and maintain judicious independence over self and environment within physical limitations.
13. Before all procedures, explain purpose and technique in understandable terms.

14. Institute all safety measures by elevating side rails and padding if client restless or disoriented, placing bed in low position and call light and personal articles within easy reach.

15. Explain condition and progress to client and family with each contact assisting them to ask questions and express concerns of the present and the future.

16. Include family members in plan of care and allow them to participate if mutually therapeutic.

Change–Interdependent

1. Medicate appropriately for pain as prescribed and assess effect in 10 to 20 min.

2. Notify physician if:
   Schilling test less than 5%
   Serum vitamin B_{12} less than 80 pg/ml
   Serum folic acid less than 1.0 ng/ml
   Hemoglobin less than 10 g/dl
   Hematocrit less than 30%
   Serum sodium less than 135 mEq/L
   Serum potassium less than 3.5 mEq/L
   Serum calcium less than 8.5 mg/dl
   Serum amylase greater than 25 U/ml
   Serum magnesium less than 1.5 mEq/L
   Serum phosphorus less than 3.0 mEq/L
   Prothrombin time greater than control + 4 sec
   Urine sugar and acetone greater than 1 + and trace blood sugar greater than 200 mg/dl if client on TPN.

3. Maintain diet high in protein and carbohydrate and low in fat or as prescribed. Consult with dietitian for specific foods for between meal supplements.

4. Anticipate physician to prescribe:
   TPN via central line *and*
   Liposyn/Intralipid via peripheral line to attain net nitrogen balance
   Vitamin B, K, calcium, sodium, potassium, magnesium, phosphorus, and zinc additives to TPN or as supplementation
   IV albumin

BIBLIOGRAPHY

Corbett, J.V. *Laboratory tests in nursing practice*. Norwalk, Connecticut: Appleton-Century-Crofts, 1982.

Gordon, M. *Manual of nursing diagnosis*. New York: McGraw-Hill, 1982.

Guthrie, H.A. *Introductory nutrition* (4th ed.). St. Louis: C.V. Mosby, 1979.

Harvey, A.M., Johns, R.J., McKusick, V.A., Owens, A.H., and Ross, R.S. *The principles and practice of medicine* (20th ed.). New York: Appleton-Century-Crofts, 1980.

Horton, J., and Hill, G.J. *Clinical oncology*. Philadelphia: W.B. Saunders, 1977.

Lamb, C. Simplifying diagnosis of malabsorption. *Patient Care*, **15**(19), 1981, 128–178.

Luckman, J., and Sorensen, K.C. *Medical–surgical nursing—A psychophysiologic approach* (2nd ed.). Philadelphia: W.B. Saunders, 1980.

39. Potential Complications of Total Parenteral Nutrition

Total parenteral nutrition (TPN) is required in the client with cancer when the function of the GI tract is disrupted due to the toxic effects of treatment or the disease process itself. The classic symptom of weight loss is not clearly understood, but it is known that the rapidly reproduced absorptive cells of the intestinal villi are as susceptible to chemotherapeutic drugs as are cancer cells. Negative nitrogen balance occurs theoretically because tumor cells "trap" or "steal" nitrogen from the body in order to facilitate their own rapid synthesis. When undernutrition occurs, the host's immune system is affected, disrupting antibody production and lymphocyte mobilization necessary to fight infection and cancer cell growth. Undernutrition also produces changes in the columnar cells of the intestinal mucosa resulting in hypomotility of the GI tract and an increase in anaerobic bacteria. The effect of TPN on the client undergoing chemotherapy is often dramatic. Several studies have demonstrated a 50% or greater reduction in tumor size when the client is supported by TPN with chemotherapy.

There are two types of TPN solutions, amino acid and fatty acid. Crystalline amino acids with hyperosmolar concentrations of dextrose, FreAmine and FreAmine E, provide proteins, carbohydrates, and minerals. Each TPN amino acid solution supplies 1,100 Kcal, and vitamins can be added. Intralipid 10% and Liposyn 10% are used primarily as protein sparing agents and contain essential fatty acids. The desired positive nitrogen balance can be calculated by:

$$NB = (NI-UUN) - 3.5 \text{ g},$$

where NB = nitrogen balance, NI = nitrogen intake from TPN, and UUN = urinary urea nitrogen.

The M.D. Anderson Hospital and Tumor Institute has defined nutritional depletion as at least two of the following:

1. Minimum 10% weight loss
2. Serum albumin less than 3.4%
3. Immunoincompetence determined by a negative recall skin test antigen

Corresponding cancers include all those causing severe vomiting, diarrhea or malabsorption of nutrients, GI primaries, leukemia, pancreas, lymphoma, and all those treated by chemotherapy.

TABLE 39-1. POTENTIAL COMPLICATIONS OF TPN AND ASSESSMENT DATA

Complication	Signs and Symptoms
Pneumothorax or Hydrothorax (central venous line [Chapter 20])	Decreased or absent breath sounds Respiratory distress Dyspnea Cyanosis, hypoxia Chest pain Confirmed by chest x-ray
Air emboli (central venous line)	Respiratory distress "Mill wheel" churning over anterior precordium Tachycardia Visible air in line due to disconnection
Infiltration at insertion site (central venous line)	Swelling Pain Tracheal compression with stridor or dyspnea
Infection at insertion site	Heat, redness, swelling, drainage at site Temperature elevation Increased WBC
Thoracic duct injury (central venous line)	Clear drainage at insertion site
Arterial puncture or AV fistulas (central venous line)	Hematoma at insertion site Bright red blood return Bruit at insertion site
Brachial plexus injury (central venous line)	Tingling in fingers Pain radiating down arm Paralysis
Subcutaneous emphysema	Crackling (crepitus) under skin on palpation. Usually not harmful.

TABLE 39-1. (Cont)

Complication	Signs and Symptoms
Hyperglycemia (amino acid solutions with dextrose concentrations greater than 5%)	Elevated blood sugar Positive urine glucose Polyuria Lethargy Dehydration
Hypoglycemia (amino acid solutions with dextrose greater than 5%)	Cool, moist skin Low blood sugar Oliguria Nervousness, irritability Headache Negative urine glucose Hypertension
Fluid volume overload	Elevated CVP, PAP, BP Tachycardia Rales, wheezing Edema Polyuria
Zinc deficiency	Anorexia Vesicular dermatitis Impaired wound healing Diarrhea
Allergic reactions	Skin rash Elevated temperature Chills Dyspnea Tachycardia Hypotension
Fat emboli (occurs in clients with abnormal fat metabolism, hyperlipidemia, liver dysfunction, or coagulation abnormalities)	Fever, chills Vomiting Petechia on chest, shoulders Respiratory distress
Hypophosphatemia (Chapter 2)	Paresthesia Lethargy Thickened tongue
Hypomagnesemia (Chapter 5)	Cramps Weakness Tingling around mouth Irritability

NURSING DIAGNOSES	RATIONALE
Potential for physical injury, related to injury to tissues and structures surrounding central venous line used for TPN administration, mineral depletion, and glucose metabolism.	*Insertion of foreign devices into the body increases the potential for bodily injury.*

Associated Nursing Diagnoses

1. Potential for infection, related to the direct circulatory access of central or peripheral line for pathogenic microorganisms.

   Breaking skin barrier allows potential opening for infection.

2. Fluid volume overload, related to a rapid infusion of TPN solutions in relation to the ability of the body to adequately distribute or eliminate it.

   Direct systemic overhydration alters fluid capacity and circulation in the body.

NURSING INTERVENTIONS: SUBCLAVIAN INSERTION OF CENTRAL VENOUS CATHETER

INTERVENTION	*RATIONALE*
1. Inspect skin in and around insertion site and prepare by cleaning and/or shaving. Left subclavian vein and site is preferred. Supraclavicular subclavian vein approach and external jugular are alternatives.	1. The skin should be defatted, free of hair, and open lesions. If tracheostomy in place, then *only* the subclavian approach should be used. These measures decrease risk of infection.
2. Place client in Trendelenburg position with rolled towel between scapulae.	2. To increase venous flow that dilates vein and to separate the subclavian vein from apex of lung thereby decreasing the risk of pneumothorax. Also helps to prevent air embolic removal by syringe.
3. Instruct client in contralateral chin–shoulder position.	3. To direct expiratory air flow away from the insertion site.

INTERVENTION	*RATIONALE*
4. Prepare solution tubing and filter. Call x-ray to stand by. Open sterile supplies, put on sterile gloves, and place equipment so that their order of use is facilitated.	4. X-ray is necessary to confirm correct placement of catheter. Refer to specific policy concerning use of filter. Although its purpose is to prevent bacterial, air and particulate contamination, studies have demonstrated that it concentrates bacteria and obstructs fluid flow. Be certain that filter in use can be used with infusion pumps without rupturing.
5. Instruct client to perform Valsalva maneuver (a) as soon as needle is inserted, and (b) when needle in vein and threading begins.	5. (a) Valsalva maneuver increases vein dilatation which facilitates puncture and (b) to prevent air emboli. If client is on respirator, air emboli can occur. Sigh during insertion.
6. Instruct client to hold position without moving. Brace shoulders or offer other hands-on support techniques.	6. To prevent piercing pleura and lung and injuring or tearing vein.
7. Assess client for pneumothorax throughout procedure—asymmetry of chest movement, respiratory distress, or any change in respiratory patterns.	7. Needle insertion site close to apex of lung and pleura.
8. Assess client for air embolism after threading occurs—cyanosis, hypotension, rapid or weak pulse, respiratory distress, chest pain, or shock. *Treatment:* Client should be placed immediately in Trendelenburg position on left side to confine bolus to right atrium. Because air rises to the highest point, blood flow will move along under it. Should the air reach the pulmonary artery, it would cause pulmonary infarction. The physician should try to aspirate it with catheter.	8. Most frequently occurs during insertion when syringe is removed for threading, or if the client cannot be placed in Trendelenburg position, or if client should exhale during threading. Can be detected by auscultation—characteristic mill-wheel churning murmur heard over anterior precordium caused by frothing of air at pulmonary valve.
9. Connect catheter to prepared TPN solution tubing.	

INTERVENTION	*RATIONALE*
10. Have providone ointment ready and preferably Op Site or other clear plastic dressing.	10. Op Site allows visualization of insertion site for heat, redness, swelling, and for leakage. Certain authors state that an anchoring suture is not recommended because it can become a source of infection.
11. Count external markings on catheter and record on dressing, chart, or other easily accessible area.	11. To determine accidental dislodging of catheter placement.

12. Regulate amino acid fluids according to the following schedule:
    Day 1 1000 ml TPN q 24 hr (42 ml/hr) using one 500 ml bottle q 12 hr
    Day 2 1000 ml TPN q 12 hr (83 ml/hr)
    Day 3 1000 ml TPN q 8 hr (125 ml/hr)
With lipid emulsions: Schedule begins with 1 ml/min × 30 min (30 ml/hr). Increase to 500 ml/4 hr or 125 ml/hr
	12. Hyperglycemia occurs in 15% of clients obtaining TPN causing hyperosmolar hyperglycemic nonketotic coma without treatment. Risk increases in clients with diabetes, pancreatitis and liver disease and those on steroids. This recommended schedule allows for gradual pancreatic adjustment response to insulin to the increased glucose metabolic demands. Fat emulsions are isotonic and do not require the same hyperglycemic or hyperosmolar considerations as amino acid solutions with high glucose contents.

NURSING INTERVENTIONS: POST-INSERTION SUBCLAVIAN TPN CATHETER

Monitoring–Independent

1. BP, heart rate, and respirations q 2 to 4 hr.
2. Auscultate breath sounds in all lung fields q 4 to 8 hr and record onset of rales, rhonchi, wheezing, and decreased or absent lung sounds.
3. Assess respiratory effort, symmetry of chest expansion, and use of accessory muscles q 4 hr.
4. Auscultate heart sounds in 4 valvular sites q 4 to 8 hr and record onset of extra heart sounds.
5. Assess LOC q 4 to 8 hr and record changes in awareness, orientation, and behavior.
6. Assess skin color, temperature, moisture, presence of petechia, and dependent or generalized edema q 8 hr.

7. Temperature q 4 hr.
8. Accurate I and O and calculate I/O ratio for fluid balance q 8 and 24 hr.
9. Weigh q AM before breakfast and compare to previous measurements.
10. Anthropometric measurements q 4 days and compare to previous values.

Monitoring–Interdependent

1. Assess results of laboratory data when available and compare to previous and normal measurements.
   Serum Sodium: 135 to 145 mEq/L
   Serum Potassium: 3.5 to 5.0 mEq/L
   Serum Chloride: 100 to 106 mEq/L
   Serum Calcium: 8.5 to 10.5 mg/dl
   Serum Magnesium: 1.5 to 2.0 mEq/L
   Serum Phosphorus: 1.8 to 2.6 mEq/L or 3.0 to 4.5 mg/dl
   Serum Zinc: 70 to 125 µg/dl
   BUN: 8 to 25 mg/dl
   Creatinine: 0.6 to 1.5 mg/dl
   Urine Osmolality: average 200 to 800 mOsm/kg
   Blood Sugar: 70 to 100 mg/dl
   CBC: Hemoglobin: 13.0 to 18.0 g/dl males
                  12.0 to 16.0 g/dl females
           Hematocrit: 45 to 52% males
                  37 to 48% females
           RBC: 4.6 to 6.2 × 10^6/mm^3 males
                  4.2 to 5.4 × 10^6/mm^3 females
           MCH: 27 to 32 pg
           MCHC: 32 to 36%
           MCV: 80 to 94 cu microns
           Platelets: 130,000 to 370,000 mm^3
           WBC: 4,500 to 11,500/mm^3
2. Assess results of chest x-ray for correct catheter placement.
3. Assess insertion site for redness, swelling, pain, exudate, and fluid leakage with every dressing change.
4. Inspect TPN tubing for secure connections q 4 to 8 hr.
5. Urine sugar and acetone q 6 hr.
6. Assess for hyperglycemia with each contact.
   Dry, hot skin
   Polyuria
   Hunger
   Thirst
   Lethargy

7. Assess TPN infusion schedule—amino acid solutions:
    Day 1   1000 ml/24 hr (42 ml/hr)
    Day 2   1000 ml/12 hr (83 ml/hr)
    Day 3   1000 ml/8 hr (125 ml/hr)
    Lipid solutions: 1 ml/min × 30 min (30 ml/hr) then, 500 ml/4 hr (125 ml/hr)
8. Assess for hypoglycemia with each contact (especially if insulin coverage is added to TPN solution).
    Cool, moist skin
    Oliguria
    Irritability
    Headache
    Hypertension

Change–Independent

1. Maintain bedrest until strength increases to tolerate activity or as prescribed.
2. Mouth care q 4 hr using oral antiseptic of choice and soft toothbrush.
3. Turn, cough, deep breathe q 2 hr while on bedrest.
4. Back care q 4 hr using deep massage with lotion to all bony prominences.
5. Offer fluids to 120 ml q 2 hr if appropriate and tolerated.
6. Passive ROME to all major joints using caution with TPN side arm.
7. Apply O_2 at 2 L/min by nasal cannula if dyspnea occurs.
8. Assist client to perform ADLs and maintain judicious independence and control over self and environment within physical limitations.
9. Institute all safety measures by elevating side rails, placing bed in low position, and arranging call light and personal articles within easy reach.
10. Explain condition and progress to client and family with each contact. Assist them to ask questions and express concerns of the present and the future.
11. Include family members in plan of care and allow them to participate, if mutually therapeutic.

Change–Interdependent

1. Change TPN tubing and filter q 24 hr or according to protocol.
2. Instruct client to perform Valsalva maneuver during catheter change and place in Trendelenburg position to prevent air entering line.
3. Change air occlusive dressing q 24 to 48 hr or according to protocol.
4. Educate other staff members not to use subclavian TPN line for CVP monitoring, blood sampling, or blood administration. (Because infection

is a primary concern, the Center for Disease Control, Atlanta, Georgia, state that nothing should be piggy-backed into a TPN line.)

5. Notify physician if:
    Blood sugar greater than 200 mg/dl or less than 90 mg/dl
    Serum potassium less than 3.0 mEq/L
    Serum phosphorus less than 1.8 mEq/L
    Serum magnesium less than 1.5 mEq/L
    Serum zinc less than 70 μg/dl
    BUN greater than 25 mg/dl *and*
    Creatinine greater than 2.0 mg/dl
    Hemoglobin less than 10 g/dl
    Hematocrit less than 30%
    WBC greater than 12,000/mm^3
    Anthropometric measurements decreased
    Rales or absent breath sounds occur
    "Mill wheel" churning occurs over precordium
    Temperature elevates to 101.0°F
    Bright red blood return occurs through subclavian line
    Petechia develops on chest or back
    Systolic BP 20 to 40 torr greater than baseline
    Urinary output less than intake by 1000 ml

6. Anticipate physician to prescribe:
    Antibiotics for indication of infection
    Zinc, potassium, magnesium, and phosphorus additives to TPN with decreased serum levels
    Removal of TPN catheter by physician if incorrect placement occurs
    Insulin for blood sugar greater than 200 mg/dl and urine S and A 2+ or greater

Recommended Protocol for Discontinuing TPN

1. (a) Slow the last bottle to $\frac{1}{2}$ infusion rate (62 ml/hr) $\times$ 2 hr
   (b) Stop infusion 30 min before oral feeding.
   (c) Stop with routine rest period.
2. Assess for hypoglycemia every hr $\times$3
     Cool, moist skin
     Restlessness
     Irritability
     Headache
3. Compare blood sugar to normal value when available.
4. Place TPN catheter tip in sterile test tube and send to laboratory for culture and sensitivity.

BIBLIOGRAPHY

Berry, W.R., and Press, H. A manual for the nutrition of the hospitalized patient. Hyperalimentation Subcommittee of the Therapeutic Agents Board, Walter Reed Army Medical Center, Washington, D.C., 1977.

Blackburn, G.L. Hyperalimentation in the critically ill patient. *Heart and Lung,* 8(1), 1979.

Borgen, L. Total parenteral nutrition in adults. *AJN,* 78(2), 1978, 224-228.

Cooley, R., and Wilson, J. Meeting patient's nutritional needs with hyperalimentation. *Nursing 79,* 9(5), 1979, 76-83.

Cooley, R., and Wilson, J. Meeting patient's nutritional needs with hyperalimentation. *Nursing 79,* 9(9), 1979, 62-69.

Copeland, E.M. III, and Dudrick, S.J. Importance of parenteral nutrition to cancer treatment. In I.D. Johnston (Ed.) *Advances in parenteral nutrition.* Baltimore: University Park, 1977, pp. 473-493.

Corbett, J.V. *Laboratory tests in nursing practice.* Norwalk, Connecticut: Appleton-Century-Crofts, 1982.

Delaney, R., et al. Nutritional support of the acutely ill patient. *Heart and Lung,* 12(5), 1983, 477-480.

Donoghue, M., Nunnally, C., and Yasko, J.M. *Nutritional aspects of cancer care.* Virginia: Reston, 1982.

Giovanonia, R. The manufacturing pharmacy solutions and incompatibilities. In Josef E. Fisher (Ed.) *Total parenteral nutrition.* Boston: Little, Brown, 1976.

Gordon, M. *Manual of nursing diagnosis.* New York: McGraw-Hill, 1982.

Grant, J.A.N. Patient care in parenteral hyperalimentation. *Nursing Clinics of North America,* 8(1), 1973, 165-181.

Johnstone, J.D. Infrequent infections associated with Hickman catheters. *Cancer Nursing,* 5(2), 1982, 125-129.

Lumb, P.D., Dalton, B., Bryan-Brown, C.W., and Connelly, C. Aggressive approach to intravenous feeding of the critically ill patient. *Heart and Lung,* 8(1), 1979, 71-80.

Rapp, M.A., Hilkemeyer, R., Copeland, E.M. III, and Dudrick, S.J. Hyperalimentation. *RN Magazine,* 39(8), 1976.

Rosen, H.M. Types of solutions available. In J.E. Fischer (Ed.), *Total parenteral nutrition.* Boston: Little, Brown, 1976.

Rosen, T., and Mills, J.M. An unusual deficiency syndrome. *RN,* 44(12), 1981, 29.

Ryan, J.A., Jr. Complications of total parenteral nutrition. In J.E. Fischer (Ed.) *Total parenteral nutrition.* Boston: Little, Brown, 1977.

Salmond S.W. Monitoring for potential complications of total parenteral administration. *Critical Care Quarterly,* 23(4), 1981, 21-33.

PART X
COPING

40. Reactive Depression in the Client with Cancer

PRISCILLA M. KLINE

DEFINITION AND CAUSATIVE FACTORS

Depression is a condition that involves physiologic, psychologic, interpersonal, and spiritual well-being of the individual in distinctly negative ways. It generally involves a cluster of common elements which are usually present but vary in degree. These include decreased self-esteem, feeling of powerlessness, guilt, underlying anger, dependency, ambivalence, and hopelessness. When prolonged, it can interfere with normal relationships with others. Characteristics observed include appetite and sleep disturbances, fatigue or lethargy, decreased motivation, impaired decision-making, and a permeating sense of sadness. Decreased self-esteem or a "very poor self image" has been implicated as one of the personality factors believed to be present in the "cancer personality." A frequently dominant theme believed to contribute to depression is anger turned inward, particularly in individuals prone to not recognizing feelings of anger. Because the anger is internalized rather than expressed, the outward appearance is one of sadness, despair, and hopelessness rather than anger.

Corresponding cancers include all clients with cancer but especially those involving loss of a body part or function, or disfigurement leading to threat to body image integrity such as mastectomy, colostomy, and gynecologic surgery. Role loss as a result of illness, loss of significant others or disruption of usual relationships, and drop in levels of estrogen and progesterone are contributing causes.

ASSESSMENT DATA

- Expressions of worthlessness or hopelessness
- Negative remarks about self
- Decreased verbalization
- Emotional withdrawal or lack of relatedness
- Physical withdrawal, e.g., curling up, sleeping, turning away when approached
- Inattention to self, usual appearance, hygiene
- Diminished or excessive increase in appetite
- Sleep disturbance, either insomnia or excessive sleep
- Refusal to see family or significant others
- Refusal to look at self in mirror
- or at body part that has undergone change
- Refusal to undergo treatment or to try new approaches to care
- Increased dependency
- Decreased decision-making
- Lack of spontaneity
- Diminished eye contact
- Slumped, in-drawn posture
- Failure to act on own behalf when situation strongly warrants it
- Failure to become visibly angry when situation would normally engender anger
- Loss of sexual drive
- Constipation
- Slow speech
- Crying

NURSING DIAGNOSES

Depression, reactive, related to perceived or actual loss, associated with the diagnosis of cancer and relapse.

Associated Nursing Diagnoses

1. Self-esteem disturbance, acute decrease, related to holistic cancer state.

RATIONALE

Acute decrease in self-esteem or feelings of worth related to threat to self-integrity and self-competency occurs when cancer is diagnosed, treatment ensues, or disease progresses. Particularly likely when the individual's usual coping involves denial or internalization of feelings, thus preventing outward expression of loss and anger.

The primary feature is an evaluation of self as unable to deal with the situation; associated

2. Body image disturbance, related to inability to adapt to changes resulting from diagnosis or treatment of cancer.

with shame, guilt, self-deprecation, and negative perception of one's capabilities and worth.

The primary feature is negative feelings or perceptions about appearance, characteristics or functions of body or body parts if one perceives the limiting of one's capabilities or life-style as strongly negative. Indicated if client's preoccupation with these changes is detrimental to overall function. Correlated with guilt, shame, and relative importance of affected body part.

3. Sleep pattern disturbance, diminished or excessive, related to depression.

Sleep pattern is so affected as to have resulted in excessive withdrawal or detriment to the individual's physical well being. Nightmares are not unusual.

4. Dysfunctional grieving, related to loss associated with cancer, its treatment or threat of loss of life.

Primary feature is the client's inability to resolve loss or threat of loss; associated with denial or lack of family support.

5. Spiritual distress, related to terminal diagnosis of cancer.

Indicated when the client experiences disruption in the life principle that pervades his or her entire being; failure to come to terms with the imminence of death and to find spiritual meaning in life.

NURSING INTERVENTIONS

Monitoring–Independent

1. Assess feelings of self-regard and record q shift by observing for:
    Comments about self, negative or positive
    Self-care, hygiene, grooming changes

2. Monitor degree of self-risk.
   Appetite—each meal
   Weight loss—daily
   Sleep patterns; time and quality, q shift and q 24 hr pattern
   Mobility and amount of exercise—daily
   Constipation—daily
3. Assess presence and quality of support system, whether:
   Supportive,
   Ambivalent, *or*
   Hostile
4. Monitor changes in communication patterns with others: nurse, other
   health team members, significant others.
   Spontaneity of expression
   Depth or absence of feeling expression
   Emotional withdrawal
5. Observe specific emotional expressions q shift.
   Worthlessness
   Powerlessness
   Anxiety
   Abandonment
   Exhaustion
6. Monitor on-going coping and its relative health.
   Constructive withdrawal
   Denial
   Rationalization
   Compliance
   Dependency
7. Determine presence of suicidal ideation (Chapter 41).

Monitoring–Interdependent

1. Observe for action and side effects of antidepressant medication prescribed for client BID.
2. Monitor effects of other prescribed medications that increase depression
   (if applicable) including:
   Symmetrel, Levodopa, phenothiazines (Thorazine, Mellaril, Prolixin,
   Trilafon, Compazine, Stelazine, Navane), Inderal, Aldomet, Prednisone, and human chorionic gonadotropic hormone.

Change–Independent

1. Insure that needs for physiologic safety and nurture are met while client is unable to do so independently.
   Stay with client in silence if necessary
   Provide appealing nourishment
   Promote regular sleep
   Institute active or passive exercise as tolerated
   Minimize exhaustion by alternating treatment and rest periods
   Continue to use touch and other comfort measures
2. Develop trust as the basis for all other interventions.
   Spend time with client on regular basis, at least BID for total of 30 min
   Accept the client's behavior at current level by speaking slowly and allowing time for response
   Listen in order to convey worth of client's ideas and feelings
   Display genuineness, appropriate honesty, and competence in care provided; share some of own feelings to show value of client as someone to share with
3. Foster constructive externalization of anger and negative feelings.
   Listen and accept verbalized anger when it occurs without personalizing reaction
   Assist client to use physical expression geared to his or her physical capabilities (1 or 2 × per shift): walking, punching a pillow
   Provide a pad of paper and pencil for client to keep daily "gripe list"; talk over list if client can tolerate
   Assist client to identify negative thought patterns by verbal expression daily, e.g., "What have you been thinking about today?" Point out to client detectable pattern of negativity.
4. Direct efforts to improve client's self-esteem:
   Allow choices in realistic areas of care that let client feel competent making decisions
   Set mutual goals that client is realistically capable of achieving and are suited to his or her capabilities; these may be small at first and can be gradually increased with each success
   Assist the client to *recognize* achievements and to experience positive feelings associated with them by giving constructive, realistic, and immediate feedback. (This does not mean praise.)
   Demonstrate respect for the client's knowledge or capabilities; actively recognize them
   Demonstrate genuine appreciation for being able to share and learn from client what his or her experience is like and how someone copes with such problems

Support coping and decision-making by assisting client to identify problems, redefine the situation, obtain needed information, generate alternatives and their possible consequences, and focus on solutions

Allow choice and control when feasible and support client's choices

Help the client handle excessive negative thinking by providing something to DO physically or by redirecting to positive thoughts (e.g., identifying the one most positive thought or feeling and focusing on it for the day)

Provide client with awareness of behaviors that may drive others away and alternatives so that relationships with others can improve (e.g., "Express an interest in what significant others' daily routine is like.")

Utilize humor with client when it is acceptable and can improve mood and self view.

5. Maintain and promote client's ability to resolve losses associated with his or her cancer, treatment, or death.

If related to body image changes, assist client to talk openly, express feelings, and redefine worth in other ways

Assist client to accept hope as an active alternative to hopelessness (Chapter 41)

Respect client's need for privacy; arrange places and times for client and family to grieve together if mutually therapeutic

6. Consult psychiatric–mental health clinical nurse specialist.

Change–Interdependent

1. Facilitate communication and collaboration by acting as liaison between client and other health team members; let them know what the client is ready to hear so as to minimize fears, shame, or withdrawal of client.

2. Report extremes of weight loss (more than 10% actual weight), change in sleep patterns, elimination, or mobility to physician.

3. Provide prescribed nutrients in order to maintain energy level necessary for coping.

4. Anticipate physician to prescribe:
   Antidepressants
   Hypnotics
   Discontinue or reduce dosage of previous medications
   Psychiatric consult
   Occupational therapy

BIBLIOGRAPHY

Bouchard-Kurtz, R., and Speese-Owens, N. *Nursing care of the cancer patient* (4th ed.). St. Louis: C.V. Mosby, 1981.

Burns, *Nursing and cancer*. Philadelphia: W.B. Saunders, 1982, p. 263.

Gordon, M. *Manual of nursing diagnosis*. New York: McGraw-Hill, 1982.

Guze, S.B. Early recognition of depression. *Hospital Practice, 16*(9), 1981, 87–96.

Haber, J., Leach, A., Schudy, S., and Sideleau, B.F. *Comprehensive psychiatric nursing* (2nd ed.). Hightstown, New Jersey: McGraw-Hill Book, 1982.

Krouse, H.J., and Krouse, J.H. Cancer as crisis: The critical elements of adjustment. *Nursing Research, 31*(2), 1982, 96–101.

Lamb, M.A. Sleeping patterns of patients with malignant and nonmalignant diseases. *Cancer Nursing, 5*(5), 1982, 389–396.

Levine, P.M., Silberfarb, P.M., and Lipowski, Z.J. Mental disorders in cancer patients: A study of 100 psychiatric referrals. *Cancer, 42*, 1978, 1385–1391.

Miller, J.F. Enhancing self-esteem. In J.F. Miller (Ed.) *Coping with illness—overcoming powerlessness*. Philadelphia: F.A. Davis, 1982, 275–285.

Rawnsley, M. Brief psychotherapy for persons with recurrent cancer—A holistic practice model. *Advances in Nursing Science, 5*(1), 1982, 69–76.

41. Suicidal Ideation

Priscilla M. Kline

DEFINITION AND CAUSATIVE FACTORS

Suicidal ideation includes either the attempt or the serious contemplation of action to take one's own life. Signals are often given by the client which can include withdrawal, depression, overt suicidal comments, statements of self-condemnation, feelings of loneliness, alienation or helplessness, and giving away of prized possessions. Men with cancer have been shown to have a suicide rate 1.3 times greater than that of the general population, whereas women have shown a 1.9 times higher rate. A suicidal attempt in a client with cancer may represent a desperate attempt at control in the only way the client knows how. That is, the client may perceive that he or she cannot control *whether* he or she dies, therefore seeks control over *when* and *how* death will come.

Certain time periods are known to carry higher risks of suicide for cancer clients because of the stress involved. These are the time of original diagnosis, during treatment including the initial hospital discharge, before and after office visits or test periods, relapse, or advancement of the illness, and, finally, as the end of life approaches.

Corresponding cancers include all types; suicide attempts are not infrequent with cancer of the breast, head or neck, and leukemia. They are also common in carcinoma of the larynx, tongue, lung, and upper GI tract, especially in alcoholics. The consumption of alcohol increases the risk factor because of its psychologic effects in lowering inhibitions. Other causes include chronic stress, prolonged depression, and excessive or prolonged hostility.

ASSESSMENT DATA

- Verbalization of thoughts of death or suicide
- Presence of the means for ending life
- Verbalization of hopelessness, of life not being worth living
- Previous suicide attempts
- Long-term depression coupled with increased energy level
- Increased anxiety or agitation
- Diminished appetite and weight loss
- Insomnia or other sleep disturbance
- Fatigue
- Loss of interest in previously enjoyed pursuits

- Lack of support or disturbed family relationships
- Presence of other major stressors (financial, small children needing care at home)
- Isolation or withdrawal
- Evasion of discussion of feelings or secretiveness
- Anger
- Guilt
- Overt attempts to control treatment (either demanding, complaining, or refusal of treatment)
- Poor pain tolerance
- Obsessiveness, overconscientiousness
- Bizarre ideas or delusions

NURSING DIAGNOSES

Potential for violence, suicide, related to fear or loss of support resulting from the chronicity of cancer.

RATIONALE

Presence of self-destructive behavior is the most urgent psychiatric emergency. It may be manifest by verbalization of intent, increasing anxiety level, an inability or lack of opportunity to verbalize feelings of anger or despair. It occurs when feelings become overwhelming that life with cancer is not worth living.

Contributing to this may be pain, fear of pain or disfigurement, lack of support, fear of being a burden to loved ones, and absence of meaning to life or religious commitment.

Associated Nursing Diagnoses

1. Anxiety, moderate, related to hopelessness regarding quality or extent of life.

The presence of high level stress factors especially in a situation not conducive to release by verbal means leads to an increased level of arousal associated with threat to the self or significant relationships with others.

NURSING INTERVENTIONS

Monitoring–Independent

1. Directly assess for presence of active suicidal thoughts or intent at least TID.
2. Determine presence and nature of specific plan including:
   Degree of lethality
   Availability of means for carrying out
3. Assess for changes in mood, anxiety level, and energy level during high risk periods.
4. Determine presence of concurrent stressors such as family or financial problems.
5. Determine client's perception of adequacy of support system.
6. Monitor intake of alcohol.

Monitoring–Interdependent

1. Observe for side effects of medications such as depression, hallucinations, confused thinking (particularly: Levodopa, Prednisone, and the benzodiazepines, Valium, Dalmane, Librium, Tranxene, Ativan, and Serax).
2. Refer the client to other members of the health team who can follow up with monitoring of suicidal thoughts during high risk periods while the client is out of the hospital (e.g., psychiatric social workers, psychiatric–mental health clinical nurse specialist).

Change–Independent

1. Provide for immediate safety of client.
   Remain with the client or arrange for a staff or family member to do so.
   Remove potential means for taking life or alter environment as pertinent (belts, ropes, curtain pulls, scissors, razors, nail files, glass, medications, unprotected windows).

2. Channel aggressive feelings away from self-destruction into more constructive means.

   Be available for verbal expressions of anger.

   Redirect energy into participation in treatment or settling of life situation problems.

3. Foster client's feelings of control in any realistic areas so that the client will not need to take his or her life to exert control.

   Provide information, as accurately and fully as possible, about the nature of client's illness and treatment.

   Offer choices and respect them in such areas as:

   Type or timing of treatment

   Comfort measures

   Foods

   Persons giving care

   Persons who visit

4. Assist client to redefine hope and find meaning in life.

   Give client direct opportunity to explore the meaning of events associated with his or her illness and the impact on life through one-to-one verbal exchange.

   Assist the client to identify and clarify his or her own values regarding life and death and the quality of life without imposing the nurse's values.

   Assist the client through open discussion to redefine hope and hopelessness according to the stage of illness; i.e., if the client is "hopeless" regarding recovery, he or she may be helped to focus hope on decreasing pain and suffering, or preserving dignity, finding meaning, or on getting through the next day.

   Help the client to readjust time orientation from "future" and its loss to the "present" and enjoyment of the moment, finding value in "now."

5. Minimize feelings of abandonment and isolation.

   Spend consistent time with client to convey worth.

   Teach the client to ask for assistance, acceptance, or the presence of the nurse when anxiety and other feelings become too great to bear alone.

   Contract with the client that he or she will inform the nurse prior to acting on the impulse to end his life.

6. Examine own ethical and moral stand regarding client's right to live and right to die so that it will not interfere with care. Arrange care by other staff if *NOT* able to meet the client's needs.

7. Consult a psychiatric/mental–health clinical nurse specialist.

Change–Interdependent

1. Notify physician immediately if actual suicidal attempt is made.

2. Administer and monitor effects of prescribed antidepressants or suitable

antianxiety agents given to decrease stress and provide relief to increase coping. Report further CNS depression.

3. Foster communication between client and other health team members, i.e., the physician, to promote client's feelings of control and worth.

4. Arrange for spiritual or religious guidance, if needed.

5. Make formal referral to a mental health professional if client's problems persist or family needs assistance to deal with threat of suicide.

BIBLIOGRAPHY

Carmack, B.J. Suspect a suicide? Don't be afraid to act. *RN*, **46**(4), 1983, 43–45, 90.

Fox, B.H., Stanek, E.J. III, Boyd, S.C., and Flannery, J.T. Suicide rates among cancer patients in Connecticut. *Journal of Chronic Disease*, **35**, 1982, 89–100.

Gordon, M. *Manual of nursing diagnosis*. New York: McGraw-Hill, 1982.

Holland, J.C. Psychologic aspects of cancer. In J.F. Holland and E. Frei III (Eds.), *Cancer medicine* (2nd ed.). Philadelphia: Lea and Febiger, 1982, pp. 1182–1183.

Krant, J. and Roy E. Psychologic Exigencies. In J.Yarbro and R. Bornstein (Eds.), *Oncologic emergencies*. New York: Grune and Stratton, 1981.

Marino, L.B. *Cancer nursing*. St. Louis: C.V. Mosby, 1981, chap 4.

Maxwell, M.B. Cancer and suicide. *Cancer Nursing*, **3**(1), 1980, 33–38.

Storey, P. and Bewley, T.H. Psychiatric and drug dependence emergencies. In C. Ogilvie (Ed.), *Birch's emergencies in medical practice* (11th ed.). New York: Churchill-Livingstone, 1981.

Whitlock, F.A. Suicide, cancer and depression. *British Journal of Psychiatry*, **132**,1978, 269–274.

Wilson, H.S., and Kneisl, C.R. *Psychiatric nursing* (2nd ed.). Reading, Massachusetts: Addison-Wesley, 1983, pp. 288–292.

Glossary

Acral cyanosis: A bluish tinge manifested by hypoxic tissue affecting the fingers and toes. Occurs with DIC.

ACTH: Adrenocorticotropin, a hormone secreted by the pituitary that regulates the adrenal gland secretion of cortisol, a glucocorticoid, is produced abnormally from certain cancer cells. ACTH is normally regulated by a negative feedback mechanism. Hypersecretion causes Cushing's syndrome and hyposecretion causes Addison's disease.

Addison's disease: Bilateral destruction of the adrenal cortex resulting in hypofunction or adrenocortical insufficiency, that in turn result in reduced levels of glucocorticoids, mineralocorticoids and androgens. Most common cause is autoimmune disease, but other causes include fungal infections, cancer, and sepsis.

Adenocarcinoma: An anatomical classification for malignant tumors that arise from glandular epithelium.

ADH: Abbreviation for an antidiuretic hormone that is secreted by the posterior pituitary gland. ADH reduces the volume of urine secreted; inhibition of ADH causes increased urinary volume. Regulated by serum osmolarity (osmoreceptors) and blood volume.

ADL: Activities of daily living, including self care activities.

ADP: Abbreviation for adenosine diphosphate, which is the discharged or energy-poor counterpart of adenosine triphosphate (ATP). ADP can accept chemical energy again by regaining a phosphate group to become ATP, the basic energy form of cells.

Adventitious breath sounds: Abnormal breath sounds: rales, produced by fluid in the bronchioles; rhonchi, produced by air passing through airways obstructed by secretions, tumors, swelling; wheezes, produced by air passing through obstructed smaller passages; and pleural friction rubs, produced by an inflamed pleura.

Afterload: Stress within the left ventricular wall after the onset of myofibril shortening (systole) determined by aortic impedence (resistance to ventricular emptying because of blood volume and pressure in the aorta and end diastole which must be overcome for ejection to occur) and systemic vascular resistance (SVR) (resistance within the systemic circulation which is determined by blood viscosity and length and diameter of the vessel). Also defined as the resistance of the arterial blood pressure that the heart must pump against and the force needed to open the aortic and pulmonic valves. Nipride (vasodialator) and dopamine (positive inotropic action) decrease afterload. Vasoconstriction increases afterload.

Aldosterone: A potent adrenalcortical steroid that regulates electrolyte levels by renal control, increases excretion of potassium, and conserves sodium and chloride. Described as a mineralcorticoid. It is synthesized and released via the renin-angiotension II–aldosterone mechanism.

Ambivalance: Coexistence of contradictory and opposing emotions toward a person or object. A conflict caused by an incentive that is at one time both positive and negative.

Amyloid AA protein: A protein synthesized by the liver which proliferates and infiltrates body organs resulting in amyloidosis. Exact mechanism of action is unknown.

Anergic: No reaction at the site of intradermal injection of a chemical for skin tests for allergic reaction or cell mediated immunity. Impairment of immunity exists when no reaction is noted. Hypersensitivity is tested with chemotherapeutic drugs utilized in skin tests before full doses of the drug are given.

Anion gap: Quantity of unmeasured anions (negative ions), obtained by:

$$Na+ - (Cl^- + HCO_3^-)$$

sodium level minus (chloride level plus bicarbonate level)

Normal value is 8 to 12 mEq/L. Used to determine respiratory and metabolic acidosis and alkalosis.

Anthracyclines: Classification of chemotherapeutic drugs which include Daunorubicin, Adriamycin, and Rubidazone.

Anthropoemetric measurements: Noninvasive methods of assessing somatic protein compartment. Depletion is demonstrated by fat and muscle wasting. Tools utilized are a tape measure and skin-fold caliper. The three measurements obtained are triceps skin fold (TSF), mid-arm circumference (MAC), and mid-arm muscle circumference (MAMC).

Antidepressants: A classification of drugs whose action is attributed to increasing the catecholamine stores in the central nervous system, thereby decreasing the feeling of depression in an individual. Examples include Tofranil, Elavil, Ritalin, and Sinequan.

Anuria: No urine production or excretion. Caused by urinary tract obstruction, profound shock, inadequate renal profusion, and acute and chronic renal failure.

Aphasia: Several forms of disordered language expression and perception. It is seen in disorders affecting the dominant cerebral hemisphere.

Astrocytoma: A type of glioma that arises from supportive tissue (glial cells and astrocytes). Is usually located in the white matter of the frontal and temporal lobes. Rate of growth is moderately slow, with a prognosis of less than two years.

Asystole: No cardiac electrical activity on EKG (straight line EKG). Can result from hypokalemia, arrhythmias, or cardiac arrest.

Ataxia: Muscular incoordination. In the client with cancer it is usually related to cerebellar dysfunction or spinal cord involvement.

Atelectasis: Diffuse alveolar collapse due to failure of expansion, hyperinflation, retention of secretions, and/or inadequate humidification of inspired air.

ATP: Abbreviation for adenosine triphosphate, which is the basic form of cellular energy. During cellular activity ATP breaks down and releases energy.

Atrial fibrillation: Cardiac arrhythmia characterized by rapid, nondistinct P waves and an irregular QRS. A ventricular rate less than 60 is a slow ventricular response and greater than 100 is a rapid ventricular response. Occurs with coronary artery disease, congestive heart failure, myocardial infarction, constrictive pericarditis, digitalis toxicity, and chronic lung disease.

Atrial flutter: A cardiac arrhythmia. Atrial contractions may reach 200 to 400 per minute, but the ventricular contractions have a regular rhythm and rate. P Waves of the cardiac cycle on EKG are characteristically sawtoothed in configuration. Occurs with digitalis toxicity and hypokalemia.

Atrial tachycardia: Heart rate greater than 180 bpm. Occurs with hypokalemia and digitalis toxicity.

Atrophy: Wasting, emaciation, and diminution in size and function of an organ, muscle, or part.

Autonomic hyperreflexia: An emergency situation that may occur in the client with spinal cord injury or compression. It is triggered by distended bladder, fecal impaction, or stimulation of the skin below the level of T-7 cord injury. The trigger causes a sympathetic surge, resulting in a reflex vasoconstriction with severe hypertension and headache. Rebound bradycardia occurs in an attempt to compensate, followed by peripheral vasodilation and flushing of the skin. Vasoconstriction remains below the level of the lesion because of the interrupted pathway. A cerebral vascular accident can occur if untreated. Treatment consists of relieving the trigger and administering antihypertensives.

A-V block: Cardiac arrhythmia in which the normal conduction pathway is blocked. First degree A-V block the PR interval is greater than 0.2 seconds. Second degree A-V block, Mobitz I (Wenckebach), the PR interval becomes progressively longer in each cardiac cycle until a beat is dropped. Second degree A-V block, Mobitz II, two or more P waves with each QRS. PR interval with each conducted beat is the same. Bundle branch block coexists (QRS greater than 0.12 seconds). Third degree A-V block (complete), the P waves and QRS are regular but the atria and ventricles beat independently (separate pacemakers) and the ventricular rate is less than 60 beats per minute. Occurs with cardiac disease, digitalis toxicity, and hyperkalemia.

a Wave: One of the three positive waves of the right atrial (RA) waveforms; a, c, and v (fig., p. 280). "a" Wave represents right atrial contraction (systole), "v" wave RA diastole, and "c" wave the increase in pressure in the RA during right ventricular (RV) contraction. The "a" wave elevates with constrictive pericarditis and tamponade because of the increased RV diastolic pressure. These waveform events correspond to EKG activity.

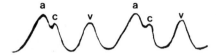

a Wave

Axis deviation: Axis refers to the direction of the electrical current flow in the heart (from the base to the apex and from depolarized (negative) cells to the polarized (positive) cells) which is determined by each of the EKG leads. The normal axis is between 0 and +90 degrees. Left axis deviation is between 0 and −90 degrees, and right axis is between +90 and +180 degrees. Axis shifts occur with ventricular hypertrophy, acute myocardial infarction (inferior), and cardiomyopathy.

Azotemia: The presence of abnormal amounts of nitrogenous products (creatinine and urea) in the blood. Occurs with renal failure.

Babinski's reflex: Elicited by stroking the lateral aspect of the sole of the foot. A positive response (backward flexion of the great toe and slight spreading of the other toes) indicates upper motor neuron lesion. May also indicate a stroke in the right hemisphere of the brain.

Blanching nail test: A measure used for assessing arterial flow to the extremities. The client's nail beds are squeezed to produce blanching and observed for the return of color. With normal capillary perfusion, the color will return within six seconds.

Bradycardia: A heart rate and pulse rate less than 60 bpm resulting from hyperkalemia, parasympathetic stimulation, or digitalis toxicity.

Bronchiectasis: Chronic dilatation of the bronchi or bronchioles of the lung. Characterized by productive mucopurulent cough. Can lead to decreased lung ventilatory capacity, pulmonary hypertension, cor-pulmonale, and pneumonia.

Bruit: Abnormal buzzing sound or humming murmur heard on auscultation. May refer to the carotid arteries, femerals, or abdominal aorta. Indicates an arterial obstruction or aneurysm.

Bundle branch block: Conduction delay between the left and right ventricles through the bundle branch conduction pathway. Characterized by a measurement of the QRS greater than 0.12 seconds. Can occur with coronary artery disease, hypertension, and cardiomyopathy.

Burkitt's lymphoma: Human DNA virus induced tumor. Epstein-Barr virus has been consistantly found in vitro. One of the common names for different types of non-Hodgkin's lymphoma. Affects children age 2 to 14 years. Develops in the jaw, abdomen, and central nervous system. Responds well to chemotherapy.

Calcitonin (calcimar): An antihypercalcemic hormone of the thyroid that inhibits osteoclastic bone resorption and lowers plasma calcium and inorganic phosphorus concentrations. Used to treat hypercalcemia.

Carcinoid tumors: Circumscribed tumors of the gastrointestinal tract or carcinoma of the lungs which secrete 5-Hydroxytryptomine. Characteristics include flushing of the face, diarrhea, and right sided heart failure.

Carcinomatosis (carcinosis): The condition in which cancer is widespread throughout the body.

Cardiac index: A measure of cardiac output in consideration of body surface area (height and weight) in meters squared (m^2), as determined by a Dubois Body Surface Chart. More accurate than cardiac output because it discriminates individual differences. Calculated by:

$$\text{Cardiac index} = \frac{\text{Cardiac output}}{\text{Body surface area}}$$

Normal range is 2.5 to 4.0 L/min/m^2.

Cephalosporins: Bactericidal drugs that interfere with cell wall synthesis during cell division. The most common include Ancef, Kefzol, Keflex, Keflin, Anspor, and Velosef.

CO_2 gap: Used to determine respiratory and metabolic acidosis and alkalosis. Obtained by:

$$(1.5 \times HCO_3 + 8) - pCO_2$$

predicted pCO_2 minus measured pCO_2

Normal value is 2.0 torr.

Compartment syndrome: Develops when pressure increases sufficiently within an area enclosed by fascia to impair circulation and nerve conduction. Eventually arterial blood flow is occluded, causing muscle and nerve ischemia and destruction. Can occur with post mastectomy lymphedema.

Connective tissue disorders: A group of physiologic disorders which include systemic lupus erythematosus, rheumatoid arthritis, and scleroderma.

Cor pulmonale: Right heart ventricular dilatation and hypertrophy due to acute or chronic pulmonary pathology. Causes include chronic obstructive pulmonary disease and pulmonary emboli. Indications include increased venous return with distended neck veins, hepatomegaly, peripheral edema, and hepatojugular reflux.

CPPV: Continuous positive pressure volume. Applying continuous positive pressure throughout the respiratory cycle so that the lungs remain inflated at end of expiration. Combines benefits of IPPB and PEEP and increases arterial oxgyenation so that the amount of oxygen delivered (FIO_2) can be reduced.

Crepitus: Grating sounds palpated or audible when two broken bone ends rub together.

cu mm: Stands for cubic millimeter (mm^3).

Cutaneous ureterostomy: Transplantation of the ureter to the skin as a method of urinary diversion.

CVP: Central venous pressure. Normal values are 4 to 8 mm H_2O or 0 to 5 mm Hg.

Cyanosis: The bluish tinge manifested under the nails and in the lips and skin due to lack of oxygenation. Cyanosis does not result until the hemaglobin is reduced by 5 g/dl, the O_2 is 85% saturated, or the PaO_2 is 50 torr. Therefore, cyanosis is not a reliable index of the initial response to hypoxia.

Cyclic adenosine monophosphate (CAMP): A substance which is an intracellular hormonal mediator. Responsible for the increase in water reabsorption by the collecting tubules of the kidney following antidiuretic hormone release. Also acts as an activator of thyroid cells as well as for the formation of adrenocortical hormones.

Delusions: False beliefs which can not be altered by argument or reasoning. Often found in depressive states.

1,25 Dioxycolecalciferol: Necessary for the absorption of calcium through the gastrointestinal tract. Vitamin D is converted to 25 hydroxycolecalciferol in the liver, which is then converted to 1,25 dihydrocholecalciferol in the kidney by parathormone. From the kidney it goes to the intestine, attaches to the goblet cells, and reacts with the calcium ion.

dl: A unit of measure equivalent to 100 milliliters.

Dry eye syndrome: Photophobia and pain in the eye along with decreased tear secretions. A complication of graft-versus-host disease.

Dyspnea: Labored, difficult breathing, often accompanied by pain. Due to insufficient oxygenation of blood, obstructed airway, inability to expand the lungs, severe anemia, or poor cardiac output.

Ectopy: Ectopic beat refers to a cardiac beat beginning at a point other than the sinoatrial node.

Ejection fraction: Amount of blood ejected from the ventricle during systole. Calculated by:

$$EF = \frac{EDV - ESV}{EDV} \times 100$$

where EDV = end diastolic volume, ESV = end systolic volume. Normal range is 65% plus or minus 8%. Occurs with ventricular dysfunction.

Electrical alternans: Alternating upward (positive) and downward (negative) direction of the QRS on EKG indicating cardiac tamponade and pericardial effusion (50%). Total electrical alternans includes alternating P wave deflection. Usually a late sign of impending tamponade.

Electromyography: Graphic recording of electrical currents generated when a muscle contracts in response to application of an electric stimulus.

Electrophoresis: The movement of particles in an electric field toward one or the other electric pole (anode or cathode).

Endogenous: Occuring from sources within the body that are not introduced.

Endotoxin: A toxic substance released when a bacterial cell is destroyed.

Enteropathy: Any disease or pathologic condition of the intestine.

Ependymous: Cancer of the thin lined membrane that covers the lateral ventricles in the cerebrum.

Erythema: Red patches on the skin of varying sizes and shapes.

Erythroderma: Abnormal redness of the skin caused by some inflammatory reaction.

Ewing's sarcoma: Malignant neoplasm of the bone occuring most frequently in males less than thirty years old. Rapid growth within the femur and tibia is usual, with frequent metastasis to the lung. Carries a poor prognosis.

Exogenous: Occuring from sources outside the body or sources introduced into the body.

Extracellular fluid (ECF): Pertaining to interstitial (between the cells) and intravascular (within the blood vessels) fluid.

Family members: Includes significant others as well as blood relatives.

Fasciculations: Involuntary fine contractions or twitchings of a group of muscle fibers.

FIO$_2$%: Measurement of fractional inspired oxygen concentration which is utilized to evaluate the effectiveness of oxygen therapy.

Freamine: An 8.5% amino acid solution utilized to prevent catabolism. Intolerance relates to hepatic or renal insufficiency.

Freamine E: Contains only essential amino acids that the body cannot synthesize. Used when hepatic or renal disease exists.

Fremitus: Palpable vibrations through the chest when the client speaks the word "ninety-nine." Decreased with obstruction or pleural effusion. Fremitus increases with lung consolidation (pneumonia).

Functional residual capacity (FRC): The amount of air remaining in the lungs at the end of normal expiration; about 2300 milliliters.

Gallop rhythm: Abnormal third or fourth heart sounds. S$_3$ indicates a ventricular gallop occuring early in diastole following S$_2$ due to rapid ventricular filling. Commonly heard in congestive heart failure. S$_4$ indicates an atrial gallop heard late in diastole before S$_1$ because of atrial over loading. Occurs with myocardial infarction, cardiomyopathy, hypertension, coronary artery disease, and valvular stenosis. Summation gallop is S$_3$ and S$_4$ combined.

Gastrin: A hormone normally secreted by the gastric mucosa of the stomach with entry of food, which causes secretion of HCl and pepsin, growth of gastric mucosa, and relaxation of ileocecal sphincter. Gastrin can be produced abnormally from pancreatic tumors (Zollinger–Ellison syndrome) causing severe diarrhea.

Glioma: Type of intracranial tumor that arises from the supporting tissue of the brain and spinal cord. Poor radiosensitivity, is radioresistant.

Glycolytic pathway: The metabolic pathway in which glycogen (stored glucose) is converted into energy (ATP).

Hairy cell leukemia: Chronic neoplastic disorder of the hematopoietic system characterized by abnormal mononuclear cells with irregular cytoplasmic projections (hairlike) in blood, bone marrow, and tissue. Primarily a disease of middle-aged men. Signs include abdominal fullness, splenomegaly, and moderate pancytopenia. Survival is approximately 50% at four years.

Heart sounds in four valvular sites: Auscultory projections of heart valves include: aortic, at right second intercostal space near sternal border; pulmonary, at left second intercostal space near sternal border; tricuspid, at left fifth intercostal space near sternal border; mitral, at left fifth intercostal space at midclavicular line.

Hematemesis: The vomiting of blood, usually bright red. Occurs with thrombocytopenia, DIC, hemorrhagic gastritis, gastric ulcers, esophageal varicies (portal hypertension), and graft-versus-host disease.

Hematoma: A localized mass of blood within a tissue or body part; a swelling filled with blood. Subdural hematoma is one beneath the dura mater of the brain. Epidural hematoma is one between the dura and the scalp. Subdural is formed by venous blood, epidural is formed by arterial blood.

Hematuria: Presence of blood in the urine. Can occur with thrombocytopenia, DIC, rapid hemolysis of RBC's as with severe allergic reactions, graft-versus-host disease, and obstructive uropathy.

Hemoptysis: Coughing up of blood or bloodstained sputum. Can occur with thrombocytopenia, DIC, and pulmonary emboli.

Hepatojugular reflux: Compression of abdomen producing jugular venous distention and pulsation. Associated with cor pulmonale, right sided heart failure, pericardial effusion, cardiac tamponade, and severe constrictive pericarditis.

Hickman catheter: Silastic indwelling catheter that provides access to the venous system for the purpose of delivering blood products or medication, as well as a route for drawing blood. Tip of the catheter lies in the right atrium of the heart and can be used for continuous or intermittent infusions.

Histoincompatibility: State of immunologic dissimilarity of tissues sufficient to cause rejection of homograft tissue when transplanted from one individual to another.

Histoplasmosis: Systemic disease caused by the fungus Histoplasma capsulatum. Involves the reticulo–endothelium system and produces fever, emaciation, splenomegaly, anemia, leukopenia, and skin lesions.

HLA: Abbreviation for histocompatibility antigens that cause graft rejection. They are present on every living cell in our bodies. The cells most often tested for compatibility are white blood cells and platelets.

HOB: Abbreviation for head of the bed.

Hodgkin's disease: Malignant disease characterized by proliferation of abnormal histiocytes called Reed–Sternberg cells. Cause is unknown. Classic characteristic is lymphadenopathy.

Homan's sign: Pain in calf and popliteal area on passive dorsiflexion of the foot. Indication of deep vein thrombosis. Once thrombi formation is verified this should *not* be attempted, as it can cause dislodging of thrombi.

Hyaline membrane: Protein lipid substance which forms in the alveolar spaces of the lungs due to radiation therapy, which destroys surfactant. Surfactant is necessary to prevent alveolar collapse.

Hydrocephalus: Excess of cerebrospinal fluid inside the skull. External hydrocephalus is excess fluid in the subarachnoid space; internal hydrocephalus is the excess of fluid in the ventricles of the brain. Occurs with meningeal carcinomatosis, blockage of the cerebral spinal fluid (CSF), or excess secretion of the CSF.

Hydronephrotic atrophy: Reduction of kidney tissue caused by distension of the kidney pelvis by urine due to an obstructed outflow.

Hyperpnea: Increased respiratory rate and depth. Caused by the body's attempt to compensate for carbon dioxide retention in acidosis.

Hyperreflexia: Exaggeration of the deep tendon reflexes, including the biceps, triceps, brachioradialis, and patellar and Achilles tendons. On a scale of 0 to +4, hyperactive reflexes are graded +3 = brisker than average; +4 = very brisk and indicative of disease.

Hyperresonance: The sound elicited when percussing a part that can vibrate freely, for example, a hollow organ or a cavity containing air. One of the signs of right ventricular heart failure or severe pulmonary emphysema.

Hypnotics: Classification of drugs which produce a sleep-resembling state by depressing the central nervous system. These include barbiturates, Dalmane, Chloral Hydrate, Nembutal, and Doriden.

Hyporeflexia: Diminished reflexes. On scale mentioned above (see *Hyperreflexia*), +1 = somewhat diminished; 0 = absent reflexes. Indicative of pathology.

ICP: Increased intracranial pressure. Expansion of the intracranial contents is limited by the skull. Intracranial pressure increases when any component of the CNS (brain mass, cerebral spinal fluid, blood volume) increases.

ICS: Intercostal space. Space between the ribs.

Idiopathic: Condition or disease of unknown cause.

Immunoelectrophoresis: Technique for distinguishing proteins from one another by first separating them according to their electrophoretic mobility and then identifying them by specific immunologic reactions.

Induration: Raised, hard area of the skin.

Intercostal retractions: The sucking in of the muscles and skin between the ribs during inspiration. Occurs with stiff lungs (noncompliant) and diminished chest expansion.

Intracellular fluid (ICF): Fluid within the cellular membrane.

Intralipid: A fat emulsion composed of soybean oil, egg yolk phospholipids, glycerin, and water. Utilized as an energy source or to correct fatty acid deficiency in clients receiving parenteral nutrition. Used cautiously in people with liver damage, pulmonary disease, and anemia.

Intrinsic factor: A protein secreted by parietal cells of the gastric mucosa. Is responsible for Vitamin B_{12} absorption. The intrinsic factor is diminished or absent in pernicious anemia.

Ipsilateral: Refers to innervation of same side of the body, lesion, injury, as compared to contralateral (opposite side).

Kaposi's sarcoma: Malignant lesions which are slow growing and usually begin on the exterior as a slightly raised nodule. Lesions are usually dark purple or black in appearance. As the disease advances edema is best treated by radiotherapy. In advanced cases arterial perfussion with nitrogen mustard chemotherapy may give excellent palliation.

Kerkring folds: Large folds or valvular flaps projecting into the lumen of the bowel which slows passage of food along the intestines in order to allow more time for absorption.

Ketoacidosis: A clinical picture that arises in diabetes when incomplete oxidation of fatty acids results in an accumulation of ketone bodies (beta-hydroxybutyric acid, acetoacetic acid, and acetone) in the blood. Characterized by drowsiness, polyuria, deep respirations (Kussmaul), dehydration, acetone breath odor, oliguria, and coma.

Kg: Kilogram, a metric unit equal to 2.2 lb, or 1000 g.

Leukemia: Generalized term which describes malignant disorders affecting the blood–forming tissues of the bone marrow, lymph system, and spleen. Affects all age groups.

Liposyn: A fat emulsion composed of soybean oil, egg yolk phospholipids, glycerin, and water. Utilized as an energy source or to correct fatty acid deficiency in clients receiving parenteral nutrition. Used cautiously in people with liver damage, pulmonary disease, and anemia.

LOC: An abbreviation for level of consciousness. An index utilized in nursing assessment to determine metabolic and/or neurological change. Consists of a determination of the four criteria: amount of stimulus necessary to arouse a client, level of orientation, ability to follow commands, and type of response or movement elicited.

Lymphadenopathy: Lymph node enlargement or any disease of the lymph glands. Occurs with lymph node metastasis.

Lymphangitis: Inflammation of lymph node or vessel.

Lymphoma: Generalized term for tumors of lymphatic tissue, both benign and malignant types. Classical symptom is enlarged lymph nodes. Benign forms remain localized whereas malignant types metastasize.

Lymphosarcoma: One of the non-Hodgkin's lymphomas. Malignant disease of lymphatic tissue. Diagnosis is made by biopsy.

Mast cells: Large, granulated cells found in connective tissues and the storage center for chemical mediators which are released in an anaphylactoid reaction.

MCH: Mean corpuscular hemoglobin. The amount of hemoglobin in each cell. Useful in diagnosing blood loss, iron deficiency anemia, and pernicious anemia.

MCHC: Mean corpuscular hemoglobin concentration. A hemotological measure of the average amount of hemoglobin concentration per red blood cell. Utilized in diagnosing blood loss, iron deficiency anemia, and pernicious anemia.

MCL: Mid-clavicular line. Imaginary line down the thorax starting at the midpoint of the clavicle. Used as a landmark.

MCV: Mean corpuscular volume. Describes the mean or average size of individual RBC. It indicates blood loss, iron deficiency anemia, and pernicious anemia.

Megakaryocytes: Large, multinucleated cells in the bone marrow that are generally thought to be a precursor of platelets (thrombocytes).

Melena: Black vomit or dark, tarry stools resulting from the action of intestinal enzymes and HCl on free blood. Occurs with thrombocytopenia, hemorrhagic gastritis, DIC, and graft-versus-host disease.

Melanoma: Also known as malignant melanoma. A neoplastic growth of melanocytes anywhere on the skin, eye, or mucous membrane. Potential for widespread metastases. Common sites are the legs and the back.

Meningioma: A benign, slow-growing tumor arising from the meninges. Usually occurs in adults over age thirty. May cause brain damage due to intracranial compression.

Menorrhagia: An excessive regular menstrul flow. Occurs with thrombocytopenia, DIC.

Mesothelioma: A tumor which originates from the mesothelium, epithelial layers covering all serous membranes such as bone, cartiledge, and muscle, and lymphatic tissue. One type is rapidly fatal, spreading over the pleural covering of the lung. Current research indicates a possible association between this tumor and asbestos exposure.

Metabolic encephalopathy: Any disease or dysfunction of the brain related to hypomagnesemia, hypophosphatemia, and elevated ammonia levels (hepatic encephalopathy) causing changes in behavior, confusion, restlessness, loss of consciousness, convulsions, and/or irreversible coma.

Metrorrhagia: Uterine bleeding between menstrual periods. Occurs with thrombocytopenia and DIC.

Mill-wheel churning murmur: A noise heard when auscultating the anterior precordium that sounds like a mill-wheel churning, indicating an air emboli. For diagnostic use: a sign that air has entered a central venous line.

MOPP protocol: A combination chemotherapy regimen utilized in treating Hodgkin's disease. The chemotherapeutic agents include Mustargen (nitrogen mustard), Oncovin (vincristine), Procarbazine, and Prednisone.

MOV: Minimal occluding volume. The minimal amount of air that is required to inflate a cuff (tracheostomy, endotracheal) so that a seal, necessary during mechanical ventilation, is formed.

Mucinous malignancies: Cancer of the salivary glands, connective tissue, cartiledge, urinary system, vagina, or lung.

Multiple myeloma: A malignant neoplasm of plasma cells that infiltrates the bone marrow and destroys bone while producing osteolytic lesions throughout the skeletal system. Has an insidious onset and occurs most frequently in males over 50 years old.

Mural: Pertains to the wall of an organ, particularly the myocardium.

Myelosuppression: Reduction of bone marrow activity. Occurs with certain drugs that decrease marrow activity, for example, Melphalan, Busulfan, Chlorambucil.

Myxedema: Hypothyroidism characterized by bradycardia, low temperature, dry skin, dull mentality, swelling of limbs and face, and raised blood cholesterol.

Natriuria: Excessive amount of sodium being excreted in the urine. Occurs with kidney disease and excessive ADH secretion.

Necrolysis: Dissolution or disintegration of necrotic tissue.

Negative nitrogen balance: Indicates that more nitrogen is lost than is gained through dietary intake. Nitrogen loss is measured by the presence of urea in the urine, feces, or other drainage. Severely malnourished clients may not show nitrogen loss until the protein stores (muscle) are completely depleted. The nitrogen balance can be calculated by:

$$NB = (NI - UUN) - 3.5 \text{ gm}$$

where NB = nitrogen balance, NI = nitrogen intake, UUN = urinary urea nitrogen.

Nephrolithiasis: Calculi formed in the kidney. May also be found in the ureter, bladder, or urethra. Occurs with hyperuricemia.

Nephropathy: Kidney disease having multiple causes in which kidney function is diminished or absent.

Nephrostomy: A surgically established fistula for draining urine using a catheter from the pelvis of the kidney to the body surface.

Neurinoma: Gliomal tumor of a peripheral nerve arising from endoneurium (connective tissue around a nerve fiber) or the sheath of Schwann.

Neuroblastoma: Malignant tumor occuring most often in the adrenal medulla. The incidence is increased among siblings. Tumor is highly radiosensitive.

Neutropenia: Lack of neutrophils, phagocytic cells, and the most numerous of the white blood cells.

Non-Hodgkin's lymphoma: Malignant neoplasms of the reticuloendothelial system that originate outside the lymph nodes. The majority of clients with this condition have widespread metastases at the time of diagnosis. Hepatomegaly is common. Some common types include Burkitt's lymphoma and lymphosarcoma.

Nystagmus: Oscillating movements of the eye as they track a moving object. Indicative of vestibulocerebellar problems, lesions of the CNS, drug toxicity, and hypomagnesemia.

Oat cell carcinoma: A small-cell bronchogenic cancer that arises from nonepithelial cells. Prognosis is poor due to the tumors highly metastatic nature.

Obsessiveness: Preoccupation with a consistently recurring thought or action. Ideas of guilt frequently form the basis of obsessiveness.

Oliguria: Deficient urine output in relation to fluid intake. Urine output of less than 30 ml/hr. Occurs with urinary tract obstruction, dehydration, shock, inadequate kidney perfusion, acute or chronic renal failure.

ORIF: Open reduction and internal fixation. A surgical procedure in which a bone fracture is held together by various rods, wires, screws, nails, or pins.

Orthopnea: Discomfort in breathing, except when sitting upright or standing. Associated with cardiac disease, pulmonary edema, emphysema, pneumonia, and angina pectoris.

Osmolality of plasma: The osmotic pressure of plasma in terms of milliosmols (mOsm) of plasma per kilogram (kg) of water. Range is 282 to 295 mOsm/

kg/H_2O. Reflects the total number of active particles in a solution without regard to size or weight of each particle.

Osmolar gap: Used to determine respiratory and metabolic acidosis/alkalosis. Obtained by:

$$Osmolar\ gap = serum\ osmolarity - 2(Na + BUN + glucose)$$

Up to 10 mOsm/L is normal.

Osmolarity: The osmotic pressure exerted by a substance in aqueous solution, defined as number of active particles per unit volume. Expressed as osmols or milliosmoles per kilogram of solution.

Osteoclast activating factor (OAF): A substance that activates osteoclasts of bone and causes release of calcium. It is the mechanism whereby mononuclear cell tumors (lymphoma, lymphosarcoma, lymphocytic leukemias) produce hypercalcemia.

Osteoporosis: Loss of bone density with enlargement of bone spaces due to demineralization of bone and a failure of osteoclasts to lay down a matrix. Results in pathologic fractures. Occurs with hypocalcemia, hyperphosphatemia, and amyloidosis.

Overconscientiousness: State of excessive thoroughness or carefulness.

Oxygen gap: Used to determine respiratory and metabolic acidosis/alkalosis. Obtained by:

$$[154 - (1.66 \times pCO_2)] - pO_2$$

predicted pO_2 minus measured pO_2

Normal = 10 torr.

PAC: Premature atrial contractions. Cardiac arrythmia in which the premature beat has a P wave present, comes early in the cardiac cycle, and is followed by a compensatory pause, as seen on EKG. Occurs with hypokalemia, digitalis toxicity, and hypomagnesemia.

PADP: Pulmonary artery diastolic pressure measured by a Swan Ganz catheter (thermodilution pulmonary artery catheter, pulmonary artery flotation catheter, hemodynamic monitoring, flow directed balloon catheter). Lowest pressure in the pulmonary artery during diastole reflects left ventricular end diastolic pressure and diastolic filling pressure. In general, pathological conditions of the heart and lungs will increase the PADP and loss of blood volume (shock) will decrease the PADP. Normal range is less than 10 torr, although some sources say less than 20 torr.

Pancytopenia: Severe reduction in the number of erythrocytes, all types of white blood cells, and blood platelets in the circulating blood.

Papilledema: Edema of the optic disk in the eye, causing bulging and blurred margins. Occurs with any increase in intracranial pressure.

Papule: Small, solid, round elevation on the skin; a pimple.

Paralytic ileus: Lack of peristalsis in the GI tract causing gas and intestinal fluids to accumulate, distending and obstructing the bowel. Also known as adynamic ileus. Can occur with hypokalemia and hyperkalemia. Assessed by ausculating abdomen for increased, high pitched, tinkling bowel sounds proximal to obstruction and absence of bowel sounds distal to obstruction. Pain and guarding may be present on palpation.

Parenchyma: Functional cells of a gland or organ.

Paresthesia: Abnormal tactile sensation such as burning, tingling, or pricking. Associated with psychosis, neurological impairment, hypophosphatemia, hypokalemia, hyperkalemia, post mastectomy lymphedema, spinal cord compression, and Vitamin B deficiencies.

PASP: Pulmonary artery systolic pressure measured by a Swan Ganz catheter (thermodilution pulmonary artery catheter, pulmonary artery flotation catheter, hemodynamic monitoring, etc.). Represents right ventricular pressure. Normal range is 20 to 30 torr. In general, pathological condition of the heart and lungs will increase the PASP and loss of blood volume (shock) will decrease the PASP.

PCWP: Pulmonary capillary wedge pressure measured by a Swan Ganz catheter (thermodilution pulmonary artery catheter, pulmonary artery flotation catheter, flow directed balloon catheter, hemodynamic monitoring, etc.). Represents left atrial and left end diastolic pressure when the balloon is inflated, wedging (occluding) a distal branch of the pulmonary artery. It measures pressures distal to the balloon in the lungs. Normal range is 4 to 12 torr.

PEEP: Positive end expiratory pressure. The pressure that is maintained by a ventilator in the lungs at the end of expiration. It functions to keep airways and alveoli from collapsing.

Pericardial friction rub: High frequency sandpaper-like cardiac sound heard over the left sternal boarder at the level of the 2nd, 4th, and 5th interspace or over the xyphoid process. Best heard by using the diaphram of the stethoscope with applied pressure as the client's sitting up and leaning forward. Indicative of pericarditis (inflammation of the epicardium) because the pericardial surfaces are rubbing together. Described as having 1, 2, or 3 components: systolic, diastolic, and/or protodiastolic. Occurs with constrictive pericarditis and pericardial effusion.

Peripheral neuropathy: Loss of tactile sensation of the skin usually accompanied by a tingling sensation at the periphery of the fingers or toes. Occurs with amyloidosis, diabetes mellitus, and peripheral vascular disease.

Peripheral pulses: Includes the following bilaterally: temporal, carotid, brachial, radial, femoral, popliteal, posterior tibial, and dorsal pedal. The scale utilized to document pulse amplitude is: 0 = absent; 1+ = weak, thready; 2+ = normal, easily palpable; 3+ = bounding.

Petechiae: Pinpoint deposit of blood (less than 1 cm) in extravascular tissues that is visible through the skin or mucous membranes. Indicates damage to the microcirculation. Occurs with thrombocytopenia, endocarditis, fat emboli, and DIC.

PMI: Abbreviation for point of maximal impulse, the normal pulsation on the chest wall due to the forward thrust of the left ventricle during systole. It is usually located at the fifth intercostal space at the left midclavicular line. PMI shift can occur with ventricular hypertrophy or tension pneumothorax. Absence of PMI can occur with cardiac tamponade and constrictive pericarditis.

PMN: Polymorphonuclear neutraphils. Constitutes 62% of the white blood count.

Polydipsia: Frequent drinking due to excessive thirst. Usually activated by dehydration or hypovolemia.

Polyuria: The excessive excretion of urine (output exceeds the fluid intake by 1000 ml or more per 24 hours) caused by diuretics, hypernatremia, hypercalcemia, high blood glucose levels, and/or impaired ADH secretion.

Precordial: Anterior surface of the chest over the heart area.

Preload: Refers to the volume of blood at the end of diastole (venous return) in the left ventricle of the heart. It is closely related to the Frank Starling Law, which states that the greater the myofibril stretch the greater the force of contraction, within physiological limits. Stroke volume depends on preload, afterload, and the inotropic state (contractility) of the myocardium. Several drugs—Nipride, Dopamine, Lasix—are considered unloading medications because they effect a decrease in the preload. Preload is indirectly measured by pulmonary artery diastolic pressure and cardiac index.

PR interval: Measures from the beginning of the P wave to the beginning of the Q wave of the cardiac cycle of the EKG. Normally the PR interval ranges from 0.12 to 2.0 seconds and represents the time required for the impulse to travel from the S-A node to the A-V node. PR interval greater than 2.0 sec. indicates heart block (1°), hypomagnesemia, and/or hyperkalemia.

Prostaglandins: A group of lipid compounds that are found in the lungs, kidneys, uterus, liver, and gastrointestinal tract that exert a wide range of physiological actions in the body. These actions include bronchiolar dilatation, autoregulation of blood flow to organs, blood pressure control, excretion of sodium and water, inhibition of gastric secretion, smooth muscle contraction, nerve function, and fat metabolism. The exact mechanism of action is not clearly defined.

Proteinaceous: Resembling a protein; possessing to some degree the physiochemical properties characteristic of proteins.

PTH: An abbreviation for the hormone parathormone which is secreted by the parathyroid glands and controls the metabolism of calcium and phosphorus. An elevated PTH level causes an increased serum calcium level and a decreased serum phosphate level. Malignant tumors from nonendocrine sources can also secrete PTH.

Pulse deficit: Radial pulse rate is less than apical heart rate. Performed by two people; one counting the radial rate by palpation and one counting the heart rate by auscultation simultaneously. Occurs with atrial fibrillation, when the perfusion is compromised by impaired cardiac pumping action, or vascular obstruction.

Pulse pressure: The numerical difference between the systolic and diastolic blood pressure. Values less than 30 or greater than 50 are abnormal. Narrowing pulse pressures occur with cardiac tamponade and widening pulse pressures occur with increased intracranial pressure and septic shock.

Pulsus alternans: Regular pulse intervals with alternating weak and strong beats; unpalpable pulse during inspiration. Associated with left ventricular failure and superior vena cava syndrome.

Pulsus paradoxus: A fall in the systolic blood pressure during inspiration greater than 10 torr. Normally the fall is no more than 8 torr. At full inspiration cardiac output is decreased due to the interference in the filling of the left ventricle. Occurs with cardiac tamponade, constrictive pericarditis, chronic renal failure, and COPD.

Purines: Constituents of nucleic acids that form DNA and RNA and from which uric acid is derived. Foods with high purine content include alcohol, whole milk, organ meats, scallops, creamed cottage cheese, asparagus, peas, cauliflower, mushrooms, spinach, potato chips, whole grain breads, bouillion, and wild game.

Purpura: Spontaneous extravasation of blood from capillaries into the skin, mucous membranes, and serous membranes. Petechiae and ecchymoses are forms of purpura.

PVC: Premature ventricular contraction. Cardiac arrhythmia in which the premature beat comes early in the cardiac cycle and is followed by a compensatory pause. The QRS is wide (greater than 0.12 sec) and bizare in appearance and the T wave is in the opposite direction. Indicates ventricular excitability and can lead to lethal arrhythmias. Occurs with hypokalemia, digitalis toxicity, myocardial infarction or ischemia, and hypomagnesemia.

Pyelostomy: An incision is made into the pelvis of the kidney and a tube is inserted to divert the flow of urine.

Pyemia: An invasive form of general septicemia in which bacteria from a primary site grow in distant organs such as the brain, kidney, lung, or heart.

Radicular: Refers to the origin of pain in a nerve root or along a segment of a dermatone.

Recall antigens: The capability of T lymphocytes to remember an antigen that the person has previously encountered, e.g., in a delayed hypersensitivity skin test. Diminished hypersensitivity is seen in leukemia, Hodgkin's disease, and acute infection.

Reciprocal changes: Changes in the EKG that occur in leads opposite the damage. Indicative changes refer to changes in the EKG in leads facing the damage.

Resorption: Demineralization of the bone resulting from metastasis, prolonged immobilization, high concentration of PTH found in some tumors, prostaglandins, and osteoclast activating factors.

Ret: A roentgen is a standard unit of exposure. Applicable to gamma rays and x-rays.

Romberg test: Tests the ability of a person to stand with feet together and eyes closed. Client with cerebellar dysfunction will fall toward affected side.

ROME: Range of motion exercises during which a joint is moved through full range of motion, which will vary according to client needs. Movement may be active, passive, or active-assistive.

Schilling's test: Diagnostic test for the malabsorption or deficiency of vitamin B_{12} (pernicious anemia). Radioactive vitamin B_{12} is given both before and after administration of the intrinsic factor that is normally required for its absorption. The urinary excretion of the vitamin is measured.

Sclerosing agents: Drugs causing scarring or hardening which have irritant properties as well as cytotoxic activity. Instilled into the pleural cavity as a method of treating pleural effusions. These agents include nitrogen mustard, 5-FU, bleomycin, tetracycline.

Seminoma: A highly radiosensitive malignant tumor of the testis.

Sinus tachycardia: Heart rate 100 to 180 bpm. Occurs abnormally from multiple causes.

SOB: Abbreviation of shortness of breath. Indicates a shortened interval between inspirations. Client appears to be out of breath, especially with activity. Not to be confused with dyspnea (labored breathing).

Spacticity: Muscular rigidity or involuntary continuous muscle contractions.

Specific gravity of urine: Measurement of the concentration of urine. Normal range is 1.010 to 1.040. The more concentrated the urine the higher the number. False readings occur if protein, glucose, or dye are in the urine. Elevated specific gravity is associated with SIADH, dehydration, stress, and trauma. Decreased reading is associated with diuretic therapy and diabetes insipidus.

Steatorrhea: Malabsorption of fat characterized by the passage of pale, bulky, greasy stools, usually due to a lack of bile. Seen in malabsorption syndrome, pancreatitis, lactase deficiency, and celiac disease.

Stridor: High-pitched, noisy respiration; a sign of respiratory obstruction.

Stroke volume: The amount of blood which is ejected by the left ventricle during systole. The average stroke volume is 60 to 130 ml/beat.

ST segment depression: ST segment extends from the beginning of the S to the end of T wave of the cardiac cycle of the EKG. A depressed ST segment means that it is below baseline at the isoelectric line. Occurs with hypokalemia, myocardial injury (in leads I, AVL), hyperkalemia, and pulmonary emboli.

Subcutaneous emphysema: Crackling sounds, similar to rales, that are caused by air entering into soft tissue, e.g., around chest tube insertion site.

Supracostal retractions: Sucking in of the muscles and skin above the clavicle during inspiration. Occurs with stiff (noncompliant) lungs and diminished chest expansion.

Supraventricular tachycardia: Cardiac arrhythmia originating above the bifurcation of the bundle of His. Characterized by rapid rate, regular rhythm, and narrow QRS. Includes atrial tachycardia and nodal tachycardia. Occurs in a variety of cardiac conditions.

SVR: Systemic vascular resistance. Resistance within the systemic circulation that is determined by blood viscosity and length and diameter of the vessel. The SVR is greatest when viscous blood is propelled through a long, narrow vessel. SVR and aortic impedance are determinants of afterload. Calculated by:

$$SVR = \frac{(MAP - RAP) \times 79.9}{CO}$$

where MAP = mean arterial pressure; RAP = right arterial pressure; and CO = cardiac output. Normal range is 800 to 1200 dynes, or less than 20 units.

Swan Ganz catheter: A flow–directed catheter with a balloon tip introduced into the brachial or femoral vein and advanced into the pulmonary artery to measure right atrial pressure (RAP), right ventricular pressure (RVP), pulmonary artery systolic and diastolic pressure (PASP, PADP), and capillary wedge pressure (PCWP).

Tachypnea: Abnormal increase in respiratory rate; can be accompanied by dyspnea. Frequently seen with high fever, respiratory alkalosis, cardiac conditions, and respiratory infections.

Tentorial notch: Membranous indentation which divides the brain into two compartments. Forcing of the brain tissue through this notch due to an expanding mass, lesion, or swelling complicates increasing intracranial pressure and creates a life-threatening problem.

Thiazide diuretics: Synthetic drugs related to the sulfonamides. Their primary action is inhibition of sodium reabsorption. The most common are chlorothiazide (Diuril), chlorthalidone (Hygroton), and hydrochlorothiazide (Esidrex, Hydrodiuril).

Tidal volume: The volume of gas inspired and expired during each normal respiratory cycle.

Tinel's sign: A compression on or tapping of the median nerve of the wrist results in carpal tunnel syndrome, related to amyloidosis. Associated with multiple myeloma.

Tonic: Continuous or sustained contraction of muscles.

Torr: A pressure measurement named after the founder of the mercury barometer, Evangelista Torricella, in 1644. By definition 1 torr is equal to 1 mm Hg.

T wave inversion: The T wave of the cardiac cycle on EKG represents ventricular repolarization. Normally, it is upright in all leads except AVR and varies in Leads III, VI-3. Inversion (upside down) occurs with hypokalemia, myocardial ischemia, and pulmonary emboli.

Type I hypersensitivity reaction: Common anaphylactoid reaction that occurs only in persons who are highly sensitized from previous exposure to low dose antigens. A humoral immunity reaction associated with IgE antibody.

Uncal herniation: Increasing intracranial pressure compresses the brain structures and forces the brainstem through the tentorial notch, causing compression of the third cranial nerve and ipsilateral dilatation of the pupil. Occurs with cerebral edema, increased cerebral spinal fluid, or tumors. If the pressure is not relieved, the herniation will progress through the foramen magnum, resulting in coma and death.

Unloading medications: Drugs that decrease preload and/or afterload.

Uremia: Syndrome associated with end stage renal disease (chronic renal failure). Characterized by increased BUN, creatinine, hyperkalemia, fluid volume overload, and hypernatremia.

Ureterostomy: Formation of a permanent fistula, usually using a catheter through which the ureter discharges urine.

Uticaria: A skin eruption characterized by circumscribed, smooth, itchy, raised wheals that are either redder or paler than the surrounding skin. They develop suddenly, last a few days, and disappear.

U wave: Occurs in the cardiac cycle on EKG between the T wave and P wave. Diagnostic of hypokalemia. Can occur as a normal variation in the presence of normal serum potassium levels.

Ventricular dilatation: Enlarged cardiac ventricles due to overloading. A reversible process if the underlying pathology is relieved.

Ventricular fibrillation: Cardiac arrhythmia characterized by an uncoordinated, chaotic contraction of the ventricles caused by hypokalemia, acute myocardial infarction, or ventricular tachycardia. Constitutes a cardiac emergency requiring electrical defibrillation. Can occur with cardiac disease, hypomagnesemia, hypokalemia, and hyperkalemia.

Ventricular hypertrophy: Irreversible, enlarged myocardial cells resulting from prolonged strain and overloading. Causes an increase in the amplitude and duration of electrical activity on EKG. Occurs with hypertension, cardiomyopathy, valvular stenosis, and heart failure.

Ventricular tachycardia: Cardiac arrhythmia characterized by rapid ventricular contractions (5 or more consecutive PVC's). Can be life-threatening if untreated, precipitating ventricular fibrillation. Ventricular rate ranges from 140 to 200 bpm. Treatment consists of a lidocaine bolus IV in the conscious client and cardioversion in the unconscious client. Occurs with hypomagnesemia, cardiac disease, and hypokalemia.

Ventriculostomy: External drainage catheter placed in the ventricles to relieve increased intracranial pressure. The drainage system is closed, with the catheter leading to a premarked volume meter.

Vesicant agents: An agent that produces blisters. Refers to certain chemotherapeutic agents that can cause severe tissue necrosis if they become infiltrated (extravasated).

Waldeyer ring: A circle of lymphoid tissue that encircles the pharynx. Can swell in clients diagnosed with leukemia, causing airway obstruction.

Weigh for fluid retention: One kilogram of weight gain equals approximately 1000 ml of fluid retention, providing that calorie intake is not excessive.

Wheal: An edematous, circumscribed, raised area of the skin, round in shape and redder or paler than the surrounding skin. Usually transitory and accompanied by intense itching.

Wilm's tumor: The most common renal tumor found in infants and children, usually before the age of five. Forty percent are hereditary, with the most common clinical manifestation being abdominal swelling or distention. It is highly radiosensitive.

Index

t = Tables; f = Figures